Voluntary
Medical Care Insurance
in the United States

Voluntary
Medical Care Insurance
in the United States

Franz Goldmann, M.D.

NEW YORK
Columbia University Press
1948

COPYRIGHT 1948, COLUMBIA UNIVERSITY PRESS, NEW YORK

PUBLISHED IN GREAT BRITAIN AND INDIA BY GEOFFREY CUMBERLEGE
OXFORD UNIVERSITY PRESS, LONDON AND BOMBAY

MANUFACTURED IN THE UNITED STATES OF AMERICA

Preface

IS VOLUNTARY MEDICAL CARE INSURANCE here to stay? Will it eventually be made a part of a broad national health program or be blown away, like dust, by the wind of legislation bringing compulsory insurance? These questions are pondered by all who have watched closely the recent development of voluntary plans in the United States, the growth of a large number and prodigal variety of organizations, and the marked increase in the number of people enrolled in prepayment plans for hospital care, professional and related services, or both.

It is not easy to arrive at a sound decision on the future of voluntary medical care insurance. Opinions on its value are sharply divided. There is profound disagreement about the best method of adapting medicine and the related professions to social needs and uses. The public possesses little factual information on the achievements and shortcomings of voluntary organizations. No comprehensive presentation of the evolution of voluntary medical care insurance in this country during the last twenty years has appeared, because of the difficulties of gathering together the widely scattered material, separating the wheat from the chaff, and measuring the value of the harvest.

This book, a companion volume to *Public Medical Care,* describes and analyzes the development and present state of voluntary medical care insurance and appraises the most important types of organizations in the United States. The first chapter explains the principle of medical care insurance and the prerequisites for its effective application, the second traces the progress of the major types of programs from the middle of the nineteenth century to the present, and the third brings digests of pertinent statements issued by national voluntary organizations. The succeeding five chapters give a detailed account and evaluation of the policies and practices adopted by the various types of cash indemnity plans and by the outstanding service plans: the Blue Cross plans, the Physicians' Service plans and the inclusive service programs operated on the basis of the individual practice of medicine, and the group practice plans. Each chapter contains descriptions of representative organizations administered by physicians, industrial companies, consumer cooperatives, or community organizations, with due attention to commercial as well as nonprofit plans, general as well as industrial, and rural as well as urban programs. The concluding chapter, dealing with the lessons of past experience in this country as well as abroad, summarizes the natural limitations of the voluntary method and outlines the opportunities for voluntary medical care insurance in the future.

Small portions of this book have appeared in *Public Medical Care,* New York, Columbia University Press, 1945, second printing, 1947; "Medical Care for Farmers," *Medical Care,* Volume 3, pages 19–35 (February), 1943; "Potentialities of Group Practice of Medicine," *Connecticut State Medical Journal,* Volume 10, pages 289–294 (April), 1946; and "Adequacy of Medical Care," C.-E. A. Winslow Issue of the *Yale Journal of Biology and Medicine,* Volume 19, pages 681–688 (March), 1947.

The whole-hearted cooperation of the executives and staff members of numerous voluntary prepayment plans and interested organizations has greatly facilitated the task of assembling dependable information. To all go my sincere thanks. Several experts have read smaller or larger parts of the manuscript and have given me most valuable counsel. I owe a special debt of gratitude to: George Baehr, M.D., President, New York Academy of Medicine and Member, National Advisory Health Council; Dean A. Clark, M.D., Medical

Director, Health Insurance Plan of Greater New York; C. Rufus Rorem, Ph.D., C.P.A., Executive Secretary of the Hospital Council of Philadelphia; E. Richard Weinerman, M.D., Associate in Medical Care Administration, United States Public Health Service, Washington, D.C.; C.-E. A. Winslow, Dr. P.H., Professor Emeritus of Public Health, Yale University School of Medicine and Editor, *American Journal of Public Health;* and Jesse B. Yaukey, Biostatistician, Farmers Home Administration (Health Services Section), Washington, D.C.

My wife, Elizabeth Anne, has helped me in collecting the necessary facts and figures and has indefatigably attended to the time-consuming duties of checking library material, typewriting the manuscript, and reading the proofs.

FRANZ GOLDMANN

New Haven, Connecticut
June, 1947

Contents

ONE. *The Principle of Medical Care Insurance*   3

Definition and Objectives of Insurance—Prerequisites—Characteristics—Feasibility—Cash Indemnity and Service Plans—Individual Practice and Group Practice—Free Choice—Compensation of Professional Persons—Hospital Care—Effect on Income of Professions and Hospitals—Administration—Education on Medical Care Insurance—Relation to Disability Insurance—Relation to a Broad Health Program—Adequacy of Medical Care

TWO. *Trends of Development in the United States*   35

Pioneering—Rediscovery and Expansion—Classification and Membership of Plans

THREE. *Attitudes of National Voluntary Organizations*   55

American Medical Association—American Dental Association—American Hospital Association—Organizations of Farmers—Labor Unions—Industry and Commerce

FOUR. *Cash Indemnity Plans*   68

Commercial Insurance Policies
    History and Trends of Development—Eligibility Requirements—Type of Illness Covered—Type and Scope of Benefits—Professional and Hospital Services—Premium Rates—Administration—Experience—Achievements—Shortcomings

Nonprofit Plans in Industry
Nonprofit Plans Sponsored by Medical Societies
History and Trends of Development—Legal Aspects—Eligibility Requirements—Type of Illness Covered—Type and Scope of Benefits—Organization of Professional Services—Prepayment Rates—Administration—Approval

FIVE. *Nonprofit Hospital Service Plans: Blue Cross Plans*   93

Basic Principles—History and Trends of Development—Role of the American Hospital Association—Legal Aspects—Eligibility Requirements—Type of Illness Covered—Type and Scope of Service—Prepayment Rates—Methods of Paying Hospitals—Administrative Organization—Approval—Experience—Achievements—Shortcomings

SIX. *Nonprofit Physicians' Service Plans: Blue Shield Plans*   114

History and Trends of Development—Legal Aspects—Eligibility Requirements—Type of Illness Covered—Type and Scope of Service—Organization of Professional and Hospital Services—Prepayment Rates—Administration—Approval—Experience—Achievements—Shortcomings

SEVEN. *Nonprofit Plans Covering Professional and Hospital Services: Individual Practice Plans*   127

Medical Society Plans in Oregon, Washington, and Hawaii
Plans for Low-Income Farm Families
History and Trends of Development—Eligibility Re-

Contents

quirements—Type of Illness Covered—Type and Scope of Service—Organization of Professional and Hospital Services—Organization of Payment—Administration—Experience—Achievements—Shortcomcomings

Experimental Rural Health Programs

EIGHT. *Group Practice Plans*   148

History and Trends of Development—Legal Aspects—Eligibility Requirements—Type of Illness Covered—Type and Scope of Service—Organization of Professional Services—Organization of Hospital Care—Prepayment Rates—Administration

Examples of Industrial Plans
Examples of Cooperatives Outside Industry
Examples of Physician-Controlled Plans
The Health Insurance Plan of Greater New York
Experience and Appraisal
   Experience—Achievements—Shortcomings

NINE. *Limitations and Potentialities of Voluntary Plans*   188

Methods of Measurement—Limitations—Potentialities

Bibliographical Notes   205

Index   219

Voluntary
Medical Care Insurance
in the United States

Every citizen may freely speak, write and publish his sentiments on all subjects, being responsible for the abuse of that liberty.
—*Constitution of the State of Connecticut, 1818*

ONE

The Principle of Medical Care Insurance

About two and a half thousand years ago it happened that Gautama Siddhartha, the founder of Buddhism, was struck by the sight of an impoverished ailing man. The prince asked his charioteer, Channa:

>And are there others, are there many thus?
>Or might it be to me as now with him?
>Great Lord! answered the charioteer, this comes
>In many forms to all men; griefs and wounds,
>Sickness and tetters, palsies, leprosies,
>Hot fevers, watery wastings, issues, blains
>Befall all flesh and enter everywhere.
>Come such ills unobserved? the Prince inquired.
>And Channa said, Like the sly snake they come
>That stings unseen, like the striped murderer,
>Who waits to spring from the Karunda bush,
>Hiding beside the jungle path; or like
>The lightning, striking these and sparing those,
>As chance may send.
>Then all men live in fear?
>So live they, Prince!
>And none can say, I sleep
>Happy and whole to-night, and so shall wake?
>None say it.[1]

In 1832, Seth Luther, observing that it had become fashionable in the United States of America "to cry out about *national* glory, *national* wealth, march of improvement, march of intellect," reproached "some of our statesmen, capitalists, and monopolists" for taking very broad and lofty views of these subjects. "They *appear* not to *trouble* themselves about the miseries of the poor. It seems . . .

> The bitter tears that sickness or misfortune
> Cause to flow, ne'er warmed the *ice*
> Of their *obdurate* hearts." [2]

About one hundred years later an automobile worker in Detroit, Michigan, head of a family of four with an annual income of $1,800, poignantly remarked: "If I get sick I go broke paying the hospitals and doctors. Then I worry so that I get sick again." In 1945, the wife of an Arkansas farmer cried desperately: "Is there nothing we can do so that we don't have the dread in the back of our minds always that if any of us get sick, paying doctors' bills might set us back for years?" The principal of a high school in Connecticut said: "Family health is one of the greatest worries of the people around here. Take my own case. Last year I slipped on the icy road and broke my wrist. Next, my daughter had to have her tonsils out, and then came the real blow—my wife needed a big operation. Our doctors were awfully considerate. But I had to pay them $350 and the hospital $125 above what I received from my insurance. I took a loan from the bank to settle my debts. There are plenty of forgotten men and women when it comes to health service, believe me."

The Indian prince who fled from his palace and forsook his wife and child in order to attain assurance of redemption, the New England labor leader who compassionately fought against the evils of the new industrialism and for social equality, the Michigan worker, the Arkansas farmer's wife, and the Yankee from Connecticut who had experienced the privation resulting from illness—they all express sentiments and state facts bearing on the principle of medical care insurance. The stories tell of fear of disease "striking these and sparing those," of anxiety over economic insecurity due to illness, of the need

The Principle

for social action to prevent hardship to the individual, the family, and the community.

No one can tell when he will be sick, how often, or how long. But even superficial observation of the events in a small community shows everybody that in any one year most of the people seek some medical attention for minor illness or injury, many need a limited amount of service for serious conditions once, and a few require much medical care, either for repeated acute illnesses or for one sickness of long duration. Over a period of years all but a few persons are likely to be hit by the disaster of grave disease or accident.

Slight illness involving small costs is not much of a problem to self-supporting people. Serious illness spells danger to the family budget at all but the highest income levels. Large costs may fall on small purses, as disease and accident are no respecters of financial resources. In any one year a small proportion of all families is certain to incur obligations of catastrophic proportions—costs wiping out a life's savings, burdening the families with debts for years to come, forcing them to curtail their standard of living, or making them dependent. Sooner or later almost every family will be imperiled in its economic independence by high expenditures for professional and hospital services and the deprivations which incapacitating illness entails. The variations in charges for medical care and their implications are illustrated by the findings of the Committee on the Costs of Medical Care. Of 8,581 families studied, 58 per cent incurred 18 per cent of the total charges, 32 per cent incurred 41 per cent, and 10 per cent incurred 41 per cent.[3] If the breadwinner is disabled by sickness or injury, loss of the wages upon which the family is dependent aggravates the situation. Time and again it has become apparent that the individual savings of the majority of the people are insufficient to provide satisfactory protection against the economic hazard of ill-health. In the words of the common man: "You can set aside a nest egg for a rainy day but you can't save for a cloudburst."

The unpredictability of the individual case of illness, its nature, occurrence, severity, and duration, and, following from this, the unpredictability of the type, amount, period, and cost of the services that may be needed make it impossible for an individual to budget his medical care costs and the loss of earnings incident to disabling illness.

Fear of want due to illness can be averted to a large degree and the economic risks arising out of illness can be reduced, if not removed. The method best suited to the attainment of these ends is insurance—the very device long used by civilized man to protect himself against many other contingencies of life.

Definition and objectives of insurance.—Insurance against the economic hazards of sickness, injury, and maternity is a method of pooling risks and resources to budget and pay the cost of medical care, compensate for loss of earnings due to disability, or fulfill both these functions. According to its principal objectives it may be "medical care insurance," "disability insurance," or a combination of both. The widely used generic term "health insurance" lends itself to misinterpretation and therefore should be replaced by the specific terminology whenever feasible.

By proper application of the principle of insurance, the costs incident to sickness, injury, and maternity can be made predictable, budgetable, and less burdensome for the individual. Moreover, access to available services can be facilitated, as the purchasing power of all those who are insured is increased.

Prerequisites.—To be insurable a hazard must be (1) accidental (a loss must be neither necessary nor impossible), (2) sporadic, (3) expected neither too frequently nor too rarely, and (4) statistically measurable and computable, or at least, estimable.[4] Even if only some of these elements are present, the principle of insurance can be applied successfully. The same rules govern establishment and operation of plans insuring people against the economic hazard of sickness, injury, and maternity.

Like any other form of insurance, medical care insurance rests on the mathematical theory of probabilities, originally designed to determine the chances of the game of dice and later, with full development, widely applied to life contingencies and social problems. The "magic of averages," so frequently mentioned in popular writings on this field, is anything but a mystery.

The probable frequency and severity of many types of illness can be fairly well measured and predicted for large groups of people and over periods of time—unless all calculations are temporarily upset by severe epidemics. The services required to meet the needs of a large group of people can be defined in terms of averages, and the type and number of needed personnel and institutional facilities can be determined accordingly. This knowledge renders it possible to estimate, with a reasonable degree of accuracy, the average amount of money each member of a group has to pay in order to obtain protection against certain costs of medical care.

To achieve effective pooling of risks and resources, two requirements must be met. Many people must band together under a single plan, and each member of the group must make small regular prepayments into a common fund. Thus the risks are shared and the costs are spread over groups of people and periods of time. Large size of the group and sufficient prepayments are essential to both the establishment and the successful operation of a medical care insurance plan. Even a large group may be composed of persons constituting unfavorable risks because of their poor health conditions. Adverse selection of risks can best be avoided by inclusion of many and varied groups representing a cross section of the population and by acceptance of subscribers regardless of income. The greater the number of persons covered by the plan and the more diverse the occupational and economic groups represented in the membership, the better the chances of spreading the risks, increasing the income from prepayments, keeping the rates within reasonable limits, providing for broad scope of service, and paying adequate compensation to the participating members of the professions and the hospitals.

Characteristics.—Medical care insurance is distinguished by several characteristics. It is a modern form of social action substituting solidarity for individual effort and certainty for uncertainty. It is organized self-help to remove, or reduce, the financial burden which may arise from sickness, injury, or maternity. People can budget and pay for the cost of medical care when they are healthy and earning. They can obtain service to prevent illness and disability and receive treatment when they are sick.

The members of the plan pay for their own care; they don't "get something for nothing." They are entitled to any or all of the benefits covered by their prepayments without investigation into their economic conditions and without obligation to repay the costs. Equal advantages are offered to all who are eligible, regardless of their social and economic status. Hence the popular appeal of insurance plans.

Feasibility.—Because it is a device for pooling risks and resources, medical care insurance is limited in applicability. It is unsuited to cope with such catastrophes as widespread and severe epidemics. It cannot meet all the needs arising out of serious and prolonged sickness, such as mental illness and tuberculosis, as the incidence and severity of such conditions are hard to predict, the probability of future losses is difficult to measure owing to the unusually great variability of costs, and the expenditures involved are very high. The method is feasible only for people able to make regular contributions. Even under the most favorable employment and income conditions, there are certain to be persons who have to depend upon public aid for maintenance and, also, self-supporting individuals and families with many children who cannot make more than a token payment, if any, toward the cost of adequate medical care insurance. In periods of slackening business and low incomes, not to mention severe economic crises, the number and proportion of such people is bound to increase substantially. Finally, difficulties in organizing groups and collecting contributions may prevent effective operation of an insurance program in thinly settled areas.

Cash indemnity and service plans.—Funds obtained through prepayments under an insurance plan may be used to provide the participants with cash benefits, services, or both.

Cash indemnity plans are designed to assist participants in paying the costs actually incurred for medical care. They allow stipulated sums of money up to a certain maximum toward the insured's expenses for specified professional services, hospital care, or both. Prepayments are collected and reimbursement is made according to a definite schedule. The amount of benefit may or may not be fixed in proportion to the size of the premium. As a general rule limitations are imposed on the amounts of indemnification for specified types of expenses, the number of reimbursable services, the period of payment per case of illness or per year, and the total sum allowed during a period of disability or in the course of a year.

Service plans provide members of the organization with specified professional and institutional services. They operate on the basis of contractual agreements with both subscribers and participating physicians and hospitals. Such plans may be limited in scope, covering only one or a few of the basic types of services, such as hospitalization, physicians' services, or hospitalization in combination with surgical services. They may furnish fairly complete medical care by including the services of physicians, specialists as well as general practitioners, at the home, office, clinic, and hospital; the services of dentists; bedside nursing in the home; clinical laboratory tests; diagnostic and therapeutic X-ray services; hospitalization; special therapeutic services such as physiotherapy and radium treatment;

drugs and certain appliances; and a variety of auxiliary services. There may be various limitations on the amount of care, the period, or both, or very few restrictions only.

Provision of service and payment of cash may be combined under one plan by confining the right to receive specified services to persons earning less than a stated amount and employing the method of indemnification for subscribers in the higher income brackets.

The relative merits of cash indemnity and service plans are still debated, although both have a record of more than one hundred years.

Cash indemnity plans, in the opinion of their proponents, are more elastic and more universally applicable than service plans, protect the insured against the burdensome costs of medical care, afford wide scope of free choice for both patients and physicians, and are free of features that might lead to deterioration of the quality of service. They meet the medical profession's demands that "the relationship between the patient and physician should have no intermediary" and that the physician's freedom of practice be unimpeded by rules and regulations. Cash indemnity plans, it is believed, protect "private enterprise in medicine" because they leave it to the physicians to conduct their practice as they please and to set their own fees by agreement with their patients. The compensation of the doctor is more adequate than under service plans, and paper work is insignificant, it is felt. "Abuse" of the benefits and excessive demands on the time of the physicians are prevented through the restrictive clauses of the contracts, so the reasoning goes.

The advocates of service plans stress that quantitative and qualitative adequacy of service is what must be attained and not merely reimbursement for some of the expenses incurred during major illness, as is the prevailing policy of cash indemnity plans. Organizations applying the service principle, "the heart and soul of the subscriber certificate," as it is called, can provide for preventive services to maintain and improve health as well as for care of the sick. They are able to place the emphasis on early diagnosis and treatment, completeness of care, and quality of service. They can give the subscribers and their enrolled family dependents assurance that such care as is specified in the agreement will be received without further payment and that it will be rendered by competent professional persons and hospitals meeting standards. Their administration at the local level entails less work than is necessary for cash indemnity plans which must check each bill for compliance with the schedules.

All this is beyond the ability of cash indemnity plans to achieve, so their opponents insist. Organizations reimbursing subscribers for specified bills cannot help but load their contracts with restrictions in order to control their expenditures and preserve their solvency. They must sacrifice adequacy of benefits to salability of the contracts. Free choice can be guaranteed by service plans as well as by others, but intelligent choice of physician and hospital can be furthered only by service plans. The patient-physician relationship will be strengthened if the plan members have ready access to the available benefits, as is the case under service arrangements. It will be adversely affected if the insured is required to pay the excess of charges over the amount he has received as indemnity or if he leaves the doctor unpaid, spending the money on something else. The total bill of the patient may increase because the attending physician may set his fees higher, knowing that part of the charges are covered by insurance. Under any type of plan, bookkeeping and reporting are necessary, but it is only under cash indemnity plans that the doctor must spend additional time and money on collection of the balance. Cooperation with health and welfare agencies, public as well as voluntary, and close contact with medical care facilities and professional groups in the community is relatively easier to achieve for service plans because of their contractual relationships with both plan members and participating physicians and hospitals.

Individual practice and group practice.—To provide for the services of physicians, dentists, pharmacists, nurses, and related professional persons, medical care insurance plans may employ the methods of individual practice, group practice, or both in an integrated system. In either case they may apply the principles of unrestricted free choice or of limited free choice; they may make collective or individual agreements with those duly licensed members of the professions, or groups of them, who are ready and willing to serve according to the terms of the agreement.

It has been difficult for both the general public and the medical profession to decide which method holds greatest promise of satisfying all—the plan members, the professional persons, the administrators, and the community as a whole. The difficulties are caused by the great variety of services involved, the large number of physicians and members of other professions, and the controversy over the advantages and disadvantages of the basic methods of organization, individual practice and group practice.

The term "individual practice" denotes a system under which physicians, dentists, and members of related professions practice separately, each providing his own office, equipment, and aides, with or without some loose arrangement for co-operation with colleagues.

"Group practice" may be defined as a system of cooperative practice of medicine by physicians for the purpose of pooling experience and skill, facilities and equipment, technical and other auxiliary personnel, and operating expenses if not also earnings. Under such a system a smaller or larger number of physicians and other members of the health professions work together in systematic association, using a medical center as headquarters.

The method of individual practice is supported on two

principal grounds. It has served well for centuries and contributed a large share to the present high standard of medical care. It preserves the personal and individual character of medical practice—one of the main attractions of the profession and its greatest asset. Physicians, individualists by inclination and professional education, will make the greatest possible effort to be "servants of the patients" and health counselors of the family if they are free to exercise their own judgment, practice their art according to their own convictions, maintain a personal relationship with their patients, and take full responsibility for those who seek their advice and help. A well-qualified doctor adopts a definite policy and conducts his treatment accordingly, rather than steering a middle course among a number of doctors. The conscientious, well-trained physician can give more to the patient than an impersonal group. The so-called "single fallible physician" is still of more value than most people at the present time seem to think.

The proponents of group practice fully share the conviction that freedom of practice and personal relationship between patient and physician are of paramount importance but insist that these principles can be fully respected and maintained—and even strengthened—by properly organized group practice units. They contend that the system of individual practice, valuable as it was in the horse and buggy age, is not suited to the requirements of the present and the future. Medical practice must be adjusted to the rapid scientific progress and the profound socioeconomic changes that have taken place since the nineteenth century. "Medicine has entered the loose-leaf age where knowledge is so vast and so changing that it can no longer be bound between cardboards and certainly not lodged within the confines of a single cranium," to use Carl Binger's language.[5] Medical care has become not only more complex but also more expensive than it was in the good old times when people used to say: "God cures the sick and the doctor takes the fee." The costs of complete and good medical care are too high to be borne without serious difficulties by any but the people in the highest income group.

To reap the full benefits that can be derived from the advance in scientific medicine and to make medical practice as effective as possible, the systematic association of general practitioners with specialists and the close cooperation of the representatives of various medical specialties must be organized. To effect economies in practicing medicine and to pass them on to the patient, the cooperation of a number of physicians in the joint provision and utilization of the costly physical facilities, the varied and expensive equipment, and the technical and clerical personnel is imperative.

Well-organized group practice conducted from a properly staffed and well-equipped center, such as a clinic or a hospital, would greatly benefit the patient, the health professions, and the community, so its proponents insist. It would provide for better and more service in a convenient way, serve to attain consistency and continuity of treatment, and reduce the costs of medical care for both patients and physicians. According to various estimates, the savings in operating costs may range from 15 to 30 per cent.[6] Group practice would give the physicians and related groups opportunities for professional improvement through consultation, research, and postgraduate study; a satisfactory income; alternating freedom from night calls, Sunday work, and evening hours; and paid vacations. It would go far to solve the physician's conflict between professional ideals and the necessity of earning a living, by eliminating any arguments for fee-splitting, and would foster quality competition rather than economic competition. As Dean A. and Katharine G. Clark have pointed out, "Physicians in a properly organized group are not competing with each other economically. There is thus no occasion, in this type of practice, for a physician to fear that he may lose his patient by referring him to another physician."[7] Group practice would fill a gap in the community health program by making good care, both pre-

The Principle

ventive and curative, available at reasonable costs. Its potentialities are vast. They should be utilized to the fullest—with due regard to the essentials of sound organization and administration.[8]

Those taking a different view doubt whether group practice is "the real thing," the way and the light. Some reject the idea completely. Many acknowledge the validity of most of the arguments but question the possibility of translating theory into practice in view of the fact that there is a good deal of human nature in man. If it is true that "it would be hard to find a more diversified bunch of prima donnas and opinionated individualists than doctors" and that "fifteen physicians cannot get along in one city," as has been stated by physicians themselves, how can they work in harmony in one group in one building? Free choice would be hindered. "Continuous relationship of physician and patient would be difficult if not impossible under such conditions." [9] The staff members would be regimented, lose their initiative and energy, and ultimately become mere cogs in a machine. In the words of one physician, "Group medicine is assembly-line medicine. It breeds mediocrity among doctors and dissatisfaction among patients."

None of these arguments stand up under close examination on the basis of actual experience. But it cannot be denied that the operation of group practice units in communities where there are also a number of physicians in individual practice may pose a problem. At its core is the question of competition. Obviously, the physician working in a solitary office will find it very hard to compete, scientifically and economically, with a team of men pooling their skill and practicing under the most favorable conditions.

Free choice.—The principle of free choice, applied to health professions as well as patients, is fully compatible with any medical care insurance plan, regardless of its method of organization.

A plan utilizing the system of individual practice may admit any duly licensed member of a health profession or only the members of professional societies. Those who do not wish to cooperate may decline participation and continue to offer their services on their own terms of payment. Participants may refuse certain plan members. A prepayment plan operated on the basis of group practice may offer admission to the service to any organized medical group meeting standards or to selected groups only.

The patient's right to choose those professional persons whose services he is anxious to secure may be unrestricted or confined within certain limits. The persons covered by an individual practice prepayment plan may be permitted to select any of the professional persons in a given area whose names appear on the list of participants. They may be free to choose the general practitioners or family physicians but not consultants and specialists whose services may be available only on referral from the family doctor or the physician usually attending the patient. Their freedom of choice of professional services may be limited to care at the home, office, and clinic or extended to include service in the hospital. Freedom of change during the same illness or within a certain period of time may be made contingent upon presentation of valid reasons. Under the system of group practice, potential subscribers are free to decide whether they wish to join a plan operated on this principle, to select the medical unit in their area which they prefer, and to designate the physician on the staff whom they want to have as their family physician.

In actual practice, freedom of choice is always limited in order to attain quality of medical care, discourage unnecessary consultation of specialists, and prevent unjustified changes. The bone of contention is the eligibility of nonmedical practitioners for service under a medical care insurance plan. The prevailing policy is to exclude them. Another problem is that of reconciling the principle of admitting any duly licensed physician with the necessity of maintaining high standards of

The Principle

service. Should all physicians who have joined be free to practice as they see fit? Should those who wish to perform services requiring special knowledge and skill meet additional requirements in order to qualify for such services to subscribers or for the remuneration allowed for specialists' services? The answer is obvious unless one disregards the axiom that competence is basic to quality of service.

Compensation of professional persons.—There is no innate relationship between the methods of organizing professional services and the methods of paying physicians and other members of the health professions. Both individual practice and group practice prepayment plans may employ any of the following basic methods of remuneration separately or in combination: the fee-for-service system, the flat-rate system, or the salary system.

Under the fee-for-service system the physicians and other members of the health professions who are participating in the program receive payment according to the type, number, and value of services actually rendered. As a general rule, special schedules are adopted by agreement between the representatives of the professions and the agencies administering the plans. The fees are specified for each type of service and standardized. They are set below those ordinarily charged in view of the fact that reimbursement is certain while collections in private practice usually represent only a certain proportion of the charges. The amount of income which the members of the health professions receive from the plan is influenced by both the number and kinds of services actually rendered and the size of the fees.

Payment of flat rates may be made according to the number of persons who have chosen the physician for a specified period of time ("per capita" or "capitation" system) or according to the number of cases of sickness actually attended. The rates may be uniform for all participating physicians or for general practitioners only. They represent average payments that are not related to the number of services actually rendered to the individual patient. It is assumed that some plan members will require little service and others much. The total compensation will be in proportion to the total amount of work for all patients. The income of the physicians and members of related professions depends on the number of potential patients on their lists or the number of sickness cases attended, as the case may be, and on the size of the rate of payment.

Salaries may be paid for full-time or part-time service. The annual rates may be determined on the basis of qualification, experience, age, or all three factors together. They are not influenced by the number of potential patients or the volume of service given. Often they represent net income. The total incomes of the physicians, dentists, nurses, and others depend not only on their professional status and skill but also on the salary scale and the additional perquisites offered by the plan.

The subscribers to a medical care insurance plan should get the highest value for their prepayments, the participating members of the health professions should be assured of payment commensurate with the value of their services, and administrative expenses should absorb but an insignificant fraction of the total earned income of the plan. These are universally accepted principles. Which of the three basic methods of compensation appears best suited to their attainment?

The fee-for-service method can be expected to be readily accepted by the professional persons participating in a prepayment plan because it is the very system to which members of all health professions are accustomed by tradition. In the opinion of its advocates it is better suited to the needs and wishes of all than any other method of payment. It affords not only compensation in proportion to effort but wide opportunity to adjust the fees to the value of the services. Moreover, it provides an incentive to give the best care to the subscribers and thereby

The Principle

serves to strengthen the bond of sympathy and interest between patients and professions.

The critics of this method point to a number of disadvantages. The professional persons must submit itemized bills based on the fee schedule in force. This involves much paper work—the very thing professional persons hate. If the fees are set much below the ordinary, the members of the professions are likely to grumble. If they are relatively high, the funds for distribution may turn out to be insufficient, and prorating, with all it implies, will be the only resort. Excessive use of the service by both patients and professional persons may be experienced. The administrative agency cannot help but formulate and enforce a host of rules and regulations concerning the use and interpretation of the fee schedule, the procedures to be followed in submitting bills, and the control of expenditures. It must maintain a complicated, cumbersome, and costly machinery for the reviewing and auditing of each bill, the regular payment of each account, and the professional supervision of the indication of the service for which payment is claimed. All these disadvantages combine to render the fee-for-service system more expensive and harder to administer than others, not to mention the difficulty of predicting and budgeting the probable expenses.

The method of paying flat rates permits estimation of the probable expenses with a fair degree of accuracy. It lightens the burden of paper work for the participating members of the professions because it requires no itemized bills, and it guarantees incomes that are predictable and certain. It affords substantial savings in administrative expenses because there is no need for most of the procedures necessary to control the expenses under the fee-for-service system.

This method is feasible for the compensation of group practice units, with the organizations receiving payment in proportion to the total number of persons who have chosen the group, and the staff members distributing the income according to their own wishes—in the form of fees, flat rates, salaries, or a combination of these bases. It is of limited applicability if the services of a program are rendered by professional persons in individual practice. The flat-rate system is easy to employ for the compensation of general practitioners because of the uniformity of the basic types of care but is not practicable for remuneration of specialists because of the diversity of their services. If only the general practitioners are paid flat rates and the specialists are compensated on the basis of the fee-for-service system, as has been suggested frequently, the general practitioners may be tempted to refer their patients to specialists whenever they feel they have done their share. Such practices would result in unnecessary and excessive utilization of the time and skill of specialists and increase the total costs of services under the program. Combination of the flat-rate and fee-for-service methods would make it necessary to set up and maintain administrative machinery for control and thereby greatly reduce the possibility of cutting down administrative expenses.

The number of patients on the lists of the participating members of the health professions or of group practice units may be so large or the demand for service so heavy that the conscientious physicians would be unable to carry the load without becoming overworked and underpaid and the less scrupulous physicians may give inferior, hasty, or superficial service. If the case of illness rather than the number of potential patients on the list is chosen as the yardstick, the satisfactory definition in general and the proper interpretation in the individual case are problems taxing the ingenuity of the administrators as well as the professional persons and straining their relations. The rates may be set too low to give the participating professional persons a fair remuneration.

Payment of fixed salaries, according to the proponents of this method, frees the participating members of the health professions from the necessity of chasing after the elusive dollar and of the temptation to undertake more than they can master or to accept financial advantages for the referral of patients. It enables them to spend all their time and energy on professional work and gives them the opportunity to keep abreast of scientific progress. Thereby price competition is eliminated and quality competition encouraged. The payments to the participating professional persons are easy to determine and budget. Bureaucratic controls are unnecessary, as no bills need to be reviewed, audited, and paid. Thus the professional persons are relieved of much paper work and the administrative agency of considerable expenditures. If for one reason or another the salary system cannot be adopted on a larger scale, it should be utilized at least to induce professional persons to settle and remain in areas where the population enrolled in the plan is too small to assure adequate incomes on the basis of fees or flat rates.

The opponents of the salary system fear that a monthly salary check would kill the spirit of adventure, initiative, and freedom to act and all incentive to be interested in the patient. The personal relationship between patient and physician would be undermined, if not destroyed. Instead of being servants of the patients, the physicians would be servants of the plan, compelled to perform their work at the pleasure of administration officials and ending up as shabbily treated and underpaid "jobholders."

Regardless of the method chosen for the compensation of the professional persons, provision must be made for allowances to cover travel expenses incurred in connection with home visits to patients residing beyond a certain distance. Usually such reimbursements are based on the number of miles traveled, irrespective of the number of patients visited on the same trip.

Hospital care.—Hospital care for members of prepayment plans may be organized by concluding agreements with governmental and voluntary nonprofit hospitals only or with any hospital in the area of the plan that is ready to participate, meets standards of adequacy, and accepts the terms. Such contracts may be made with each hospital individually or with hospital associations or administrative agencies collectively. The quality of the hospital rather than the type of ownership should receive foremost attention in deciding on admission.

The "per diem" method of payment is the only one which deserves consideration. Actually it is in general use. In computing the length of stay of the patient, the day of admission may be counted a full day and the day of discharge or death excluded, or other suitable arrangements may be made.

The determination of fair rates is beset with difficulties. The quality, organization, and operating costs of the participating hospitals are likely to differ greatly. Should the rates be different for each hospital, uniform for all hospitals in a given area, or scaled according to their standards? Should they cover the actual cost of service to the members of the plan or only part of it? Payment of different rates to each hospital would result not only in local competition on a price basis but in a great amount of administrative work. Uniform average rates are advantageous to the administration because the management of the plan is simplified. They may benefit hospitals of lesser quality because their operating costs are comparatively low but are certain to penalize the best hospitals with maintenance costs far beyond the average. Grading of rates according to standards requires classification of the participating hospitals, a rather difficult undertaking, and administrative work for checking of bills as to compliance with group rates. But this method has the great advantage of being fair to the various hospitals and of encouraging improvement in the quality where there is room for it. No matter which policy is followed, uniform or at least comparable methods of accounting and cost computing must be adopted by all participating hospitals.

The Principle

With reliable cost data at hand, reasonable rates of payment for all the services covered by prepayments can be set.

The rates may be paid for itemized services or may be inclusive, covering most or all of the charges for specified types of accommodation, meals and dietary service, use of operating and delivery room, general nursing, ordinary clinical laboratory and roentgenological services, routine medications and dressings, and other services specified, such as physiotherapy. The policy of paying multiple rates makes the spending of much time, effort, and money on administration inevitable and is a direct invitation to trouble. It may induce some hospitals to determine the period of hospitalization and the number of services on the basis of the payments allowed or the patient's wishes rather than according to the patient's need for hospitalization. Payment of inclusive rates per patient day eliminates these shortcomings but may occasionally turn out to be disadvantageous to hospitals, especially those experiencing an unusual demand for much costly service to persons covered by a medical care insurance plan.

Non-participating hospitals may have to be used by plan members in emergencies or when participating hospitals are overcrowded. In such cases payment may be made to the extent provided for participating hospitals or for part of the bill only.

Effect on income of professions and hospitals.—Assurance of payment from medical care insurance plans enables the participating professional persons and hospitals to give more service to more people. Receipts from medical care insurance plans will constitute a major source of income for physicians, dentists, pharmacists, and other groups as well as for general and certain special hospitals when a large proportion of the population is covered by such programs. Guarantee of payment makes it possible for physicians and dentists to settle and remain in areas otherwise unable to support them.

Administration.—Voluntary medical care insurance plans

may be organized and administered by commercial companies or by nonprofit associations created for this purpose. In either case they are subject to state laws defining the conditions under which plans applying the principle of insurance may be initiated and operated.

Commercial companies insuring expenses for medical care may take full responsibility for all administrative functions involved or delegate part of it to such groups as employers or unions. Nonprofit plans usually are managed by special agencies.

The administration of a nonprofit prepayment plan for medical care must be democratic, simple, and inexpensive. The administrative structure of all agencies and the administrative procedures of each service unit must be such as to assure early diagnosis, early, prompt, and thorough treatment, high standards of service, and continuity and consistency of care.

The attainment of these principles requires the establishment and maintenance of self-governing administrative bodies with clearly defined powers, duties, and functions; participation of the subscribers, the health professions, and the representatives of hospitals in policy-making and management of the plan; professional direction and supervision of all professional matters; cooperation of the prepayment plans with other community agencies responsible for health and welfare activities; and supervision of the organizations by official agencies of the states.

Administrative bodies may be set up as local, district, or state-wide organizations. The decision depends largely on the distribution of the functions that are to be discharged. Sound administration of direct service, including enrollment, collection of prepayments, and supervision as to adequacy of care, requires decentralization of agencies in order to bring the administrative unit close to both the people enrolled in the plan and the participating professional persons and hospitals.

The Principle

On the other hand there is need for centralization at the state level of such functions as the formulation of the broad policies governing the organization and operation of the plan; the determination and enforcement of standards for the service, the participation of hospitals and professional persons, and the management; the promotion of public relations; the provision of consultant service; the collection of statistical data; and the publication of annual reports.

The principle of decentralization must not be carried too far. Creation of numerous local agencies for small geographical or political areas spells waste of effort, time, and money. The past carries the plain lesson that district organization is the method of choice in building a sound structure for the administration of direct service. Districts convenient for proper administrative effort may be created by dividing large political units into medical service areas according to the size and density of the population rather than according to artificial political boundaries, and by establishing in each area a sufficient number of branch offices close to the persons eligible for service.

The services of physicians and related groups and of hospitals are so closely related to one another and so interdependent, both professionally and economically, that they should be considered as an entity and administered by a single agency. Separation of their administration inevitably will result in duplication, overlapping, and high costs of management.

If there is to be democratic control of a medical care insurance plan, boards of directors, elected by and from all participating groups, must be vested with authority for the administration; all groups concerned must have seat and voice in the administrative bodies; and the powers, duties, and functions of each group must be set forth in bylaws. The principal groups which ought to be represented on the board of directors are the subscribers, the participating physicians and allied groups, and the participating hospitals. Other persons, such as representatives of official and voluntary health and welfare agencies, should be invited to serve as nonvoting members of the boards in order to foster cooperation with all agencies in the community. Responsibility for all professional matters must rest entirely and solely with representatives of the various professions concerned, and this principle must be embodied in the bylaws. Neither lay control of professional services nor professional control of economic aspects and general policies are conducive to successful development and effective management of plans serving the community.

To assist the administrative agencies in discharging their many tasks to the best interest of all, advisory committees composed of representatives of the various groups must be established and technical committees consisting of experts in special fields may be appointed, whenever necessary. To manage the plans according to the policies and procedures laid down by the boards of directors, qualified full-time personnel, including medical directors, business managers, and various types of clerical personnel, must be employed.

Supervision of any medical care insurance plan by official state agencies is an accepted principle. What type of agency should be clothed with supervisory powers over nonprofit prepayment plans is an open question, and how far their authority should extend is much debated. In the past, the insurance departments of the states have been made responsible for the regulation and supervision of nonprofit prepayment plans as well as commercial firms. Usually they are empowered to decide on the articles of incorporation, the application for license to operate, the prepayment rates, and the rates of payment to the participating professional persons and hospitals. They are charged with the duty of supervising the finances of the plans and enforcing compliance with the laws governing their operation in general.

The policy of making the establishment and operation of

nonprofit prepayment plans for medical care subject to regulation and supervision by insurance departments rests on the fact that such organizations, like commercial insurance companies, apply the principle of insurance even if they are classed in a special legal category. Although this is correct, it is equally true that there are profound differences between nonprofit and commercial plans apart from their form of organization. The nonprofit plans are designed to promote a wider distribution of good medical care at the least possible expense. They attain this objective by guaranteeing service to the subscribers from participating professional persons and hospitals and by operating as intermediary agencies representing the interest of all. The commercial companies contract with policyholders to indemnify them for a monetary loss after its occurrence without making arrangements for professional or hospital service.

The problem of devising an appropriate administrative machinery for the regulation and supervision of nonprofit prepayment plans is twofold. Adequacy of service must be assured, and compliance with statutes and actuarial soundness must be enforced. If this be true, official agencies, such as health departments or inclusive social welfare departments, must share administrative responsibility with insurance departments according to a definite plan of cooperation.

Education on medical care insurance.—A medical care insurance plan can be initiated successfully and operated effectively and economically only if it has the willing and intelligent cooperation of all groups concerned. To take a different stand is to view life through rose-colored glasses. There is need for extensive, intensive, and continuous education of the people who are to receive care, the professions and hospitals ready to render service, and the personnel in charge of administration.

The basic principles underlying a medical care insurance plan must be fully comprehended by all. Everybody who can afford it must be ready to "subject himself to a small deprivation, in order that no man may be subjected to a great loss," as a committee of the British House of Commons stated as early as 1825. Everybody must clearly understand the implications of a plan that is mutual and cooperative in every respect. The contributions of all members are used to aid each member in case of need. In any one year the healthy will pay for the sick, and those needing little care will pay for members requiring much, but over a period of years almost every member will need the full protection of the plan. The financial sacrifice necessary to obtain security is small compared with the probable expenditures and losses.

Methodical education of the public in the principles and practices of organized self-help through the device of insurance will go far toward arousing interest in prepayment plans for medical care, winning confidence in the method, and promoting responsive action. Systematic education of the insured in personal hygiene, physical fitness, and the full and discriminating use of the available service will serve to encourage early diagnosis and treatment, improve the efficacy of medical care, and reduce expenditures for the treatment of serious illness of long duration.

Expansion and intensification of educational efforts will bring with it changes in the pattern of medical, dental, and nursing practice. Education in general and health education in particular increase existing demand for good medical care and create a new demand for certain services hitherto regarded as luxuries or not sought because of lack of understanding. Those who are taught "see your doctor early before he has to see you" naturally want more and better service. As a doctor in a small town once wrote, "The pioneers were satisfied if they could have a doctor only at most critical illnesses. Today people expect of medical service that it will prevent disease, promote health, and enlarge life. The public, having been encouraged to demand the abundant life, wants the good care to which it is entitled . . ." These changes in attitude will result in more calls for complete physical examinations, treatment of minor illnesses, and diagnosis and treatment of borderline conditions, mental as well as physical. Ultimately, properly organized health education will decrease the need for emergency service and for the care of patients with chronic ailments.

Inevitably, there will be some plan members who present problems by asking queer questions, desiring services which are unnecessary in the opinion of the expert, or trying to take undue advantage of the provisions because they have what is popularly called "the money-back complex." This too is a problem that calls for education first and disciplinary measures last.

To carry out such educational work, medical care insurance plans need personnel well trained in this special field of activity. Health educators can make a valuable contribution to the development of plans by interpreting the need for joint action and the principles governing the establishment and operation of such organizations. They have an important function to perform in the day-by-day work of the plan by educating the subscribers and their enrolled dependents in the intelligent and discriminating use of the services as well as in the principles of healthful living.

The professional persons who are to render service under a medical care insurance program must receive instruction in the socioeconomic aspects of health and disease and in the principles and problems of organizing medical care. This calls for changes in the curricula of schools of medicine, dentistry, nursing, and social work and for postgraduate education in these four fields.

To obtain well-qualified administrative personnel, provisions for the education of specialists in administration of medical care programs must be made by postgraduate schools, especially schools of public health.[10]

Relation to disability insurance.—Persons unable to earn

their normal wages or salaries because of disabling illness or accident are confronted with two fundamentally different problems: to maintain a standard of living compatible with health and decency and to meet their obligations for medical care. To a large degree the first need can be met by disability insurance and the second one by medical care insurance.

Disability insurance is a method of pooling risks and resources to compensate the insured for loss of earnings due to disability. Such plans may cover all or a varying combination of the following hazards: temporary disability resulting from sickness, accident, and maternity; and long-term disability, including invalidity, due to sickness and accident. They pay the insured specified amounts of money according to widely varying schedules.

Disability insurance and medical care insurance are interrelated and complementary. The purpose of protecting the insured and his family against serious decline in their standard of living, if not against poverty and dependency, cannot be accomplished if the money received from the plan must be used to pay doctor or hospital bills. Medical care insurance plans cannot function effectively if the efforts to restore health quickly, completely, and economically are impeded or defeated by the poor economic conditions under which the subscriber has to live.

Relation to a broad health program.—Medical care insurance in itself, no matter how wide the scope of its service and how comprehensive the coverage of the population, does not constitute a broad health program. It is a part of it—and an indispensable part at that. To be successful it must be integrated with comprehensive provisions for the preservation and promotion of health; a balanced system of adequate hospitals, clinics, health centers, and related facilities; and effective organization of professional services.

Full development of all the basic public health services to prevent disease and promote good health is essential to the

The Principle

economical operation of any medical care insurance plan. If such services are deficient the plan is certain to be burdened with heavy expenses for the treatment of patients with acute illnesses, serious accidents, and exacerbations of old conditions that could have been reduced in frequency and severity, if not prevented. To initiate a prepayment plan for medical care in an area with rudimentary machinery for mass prevention is like putting the cart before the horse. To operate a plan under such conditions is as unsafe as wading in unknown water.

The second prerequisite for the establishment and successful operation of a medical care insurance plan is the availability of adequate general and special hospitals, including out-patient departments, and of district centers serving as the headquarters of physicians and related groups in private practice as well as of personnel employed by public and private agencies. Areas in which such facilities are lacking or scarce are unsuited to the proper development of a prepayment plan because care of bed-patients cannot be guaranteed. Areas possessing only hospitals of inferior quality cannot be served adequately because the members of the organization cannot be given assurance that they will receive their money's worth. Before steps are taken to initiate a medical care insurance plan, two problems must be settled. High-grade hospitals and related facilities must be built where they are needed. The standards of existing hospitals must be raised where improvement is possible. The "regional approach" is imperative to the sound solution of the building problem because it is the only one to permit development of an integrated system of facilities, including all types of hospitals and district health centers, on the basis of service areas cutting across the lines of small political units. Licensure and regular inspection of all facilities for medical care are indispensable to the improvement of their quality.

A sufficient number of competent physicians, dentists, and related professional persons in each service area is the third condition necessary for the initiation and operation of a medical care insurance plan. In some communities the total number of duly licensed members of the health professions in active practice may be more than adequate to satisfy the requirements of the population enrolled in a prepayment plan, but it may include many older persons physically unable to render much service, relatively many general practitioners and too few accredited specialists, or some persons with very limited skill and experience. In other areas there may be an appalling lack of qualified professional persons. Moreover, it may well happen that the best trained and most experienced members of the medical and dental professions observe an attitude of watchful waiting toward a prepayment plan, while the less qualified physicians and dentists immediately agree to participate. This barrier to the development of medical care insurance can be removed by the provision of adequate hospitals and physical facilities for office practice; organization of smooth cooperation between general practitioners and specialists; and adequate compensation for service to plan members. As ample experience has shown, ready access to good hospitals, availability of consultant service, and purchasing power of the population are the principal factors determining the choice of the community in which physicians and other members of the health professions settle and remain. The least that medical care insurance can do is to increase the purchasing power of people by pooling their resources. Thus it can further the better distribution of physicians, dentists, nurses, and other groups.

In itself, insurance against the costs of medical care is a purely financial mechanism. But the method lends itself to the attainment of more than protection against the economic hazards of illness. Medical care insurance plans placing the emphasis on arrangements for the collection of funds from the contributors and the disbursement of money to the participating professional persons and hospitals fulfill economic functions that must not be minimized. But there they stop.

The Principle

In contrast, prepayment plans providing for proper organization of professional and hospital services for subscribers and their families can greatly contribute to the wider distribution of adequate medical care, preventive as well as curative; the promotion of psychosomatic medicine; the reduction of the frequency and duration of serious stages of illness, complications, and chronic ailments; the removal of the fear of want; and the prevention of poverty.

The value of a medical care insurance plan depends on the degree to which it accomplishes the purpose of providing adequate medical care at reasonable cost.

Adequacy of medical care.—Adequate medical care has both a quantitative and qualitative aspect, as Roger I. Lee and Lewis W. Jones have stated.[11] Quantity and quality of medical care are parts of an integral whole. They cannot be separated without injuring both.

To be adequate in quantity, a medical care program must be broad in scope and well balanced. It must provide for all services needed by the apparently healthy, acutely sick, convalescent, and chronically ill, including care at the home, office, clinic, general hospital, special hospital, and custodial institution, in the amount and for the period required. Type, scope, amount, and period of service taken together make up the inclusive concept of quantitative adequacy of medical care.

The quality of medical care depends on the competence of the members of the health professions, the standards of the facilities for medical care, and the efficiency of organization of professional and institutional services. These factors are interrelated. If all are present, the services made available under an organized program can reasonably be expected to meet high requirements.

The principal factors affecting both quantitative and qualitative adequacy of medical care are the method of raising funds for the support of an organized program; the method and rate of payment to the members of the health professions and the hospitals, clinics, and related facilities; and the method of administrative organization of the program.

As has been stated before, any plan applying the principle of insurance has limitations that are inherent in the method. Fanciful expectations will only lead to bitter disappointment. Exuberant proposals for "complete security" rest on anything but a scientific basis. Facts do not cease to exist because they are ignored. Within its natural limitations the method of medical care insurance offers considerable scope for development.

The policies and practices followed by the voluntary plans in this country, their experience, and their achievements and shortcomings will be discussed in subsequent chapters.

TWO

Trends of Development in the United States

PIONEERING

VOLUNTARY medical care insurance in the United States dates back to the second half of the nineteenth century. Its beginnings were as haphazard as the growth of the cities that signalized the advent of the technical revolution, its methods of organization as diverse as the background of the people who banded together. Wherever these people lived, whatever their national origin, race, creed, political affiliation, occupation, or income—they were united by their faith in the ethical maxim "bear ye one another's burden," by their belief in the principle of self-help through solidarity. If there was anything they disliked, it was the practice of "passing the hat" or resort to humiliating relief after illness had struck. What they desired was an organization enabling them to budget for contingencies of life and to escape from privation. To this end they founded special associations or extended the scope of activities of existing societies. Despite their widely varying names, all these organizations were nonprofit and cooperatively administered, applying the principle of insurance by charging their members regular dues for the benefits provided. One group of organizations became known as mutual benefit associations and a second one as fraternal beneficiary societies.

Mutual benefit associations.—A few mutual benefit associations were established in the second half of the nineteenth century. Some were initiated and operated primarily for the purpose of providing medical care. Others were designed to protect members from want.

Among the earliest associations were three in California.

The story of their development is interesting in many respects. La Société Française de Bienfaisance Mutuelle de San Francisco was founded in 1851, erected its own hospital in 1852, and remained active until the present. The French Hospital in that city has evolved out of the early institution. The German General Benevolent Society of San Francisco was formed in 1854, began to provide hospitalization in a makeshift building in 1855, and opened a hospital of its own in 1858.[1] Its successor, the Franklin General Benevolent Society, continues to own and maintain a general hospital, the Franklin Hospital, and to operate a prepayment plan covering professional services and hospitalization. La Société Française de Bienfaisance Mutuelle de Los Angeles was founded in 1860. By 1869 it had 300 members and a capital of $10,000. With this money it bought land and built a hospital (Maison de Santé), which opened in 1870. A document placed in the cornerstone admonished all who at some future day would read it to follow the example of the French, "Let them unite to succor and relieve the distressed."[2] In 1884 this organization had 551 members and provided hospitalization for 61 and home care for 246 persons. It disappeared soon after, but the French Hospital still exists.[3]

In the latter part of the nineteenth century, mutual benefit associations developed primarily in industrial and business firms. Some were initiated and administered by the employees, others by the employers, and an increasing number by both together. They were financed by dues of the employee-members only, by joint contributions of the companies and employees, or, in a few instances, entirely by the companies. Not infrequently special assessments were made when the funds ran low. Payment of limited amounts of cash benefits in case of disability ("sickness benefits") and death ("death benefits") was the primary purpose of all the associations. Provisions for some medical care were rare. To carry out their functions these societies employed physicians for certification of disability and for medical advice to the members. Often this was the beginning of an organized medical care program. Telling is the story of the Macy Mutual Aid Association.

The Macy Mutual Aid Association was founded in 1885 by a group of employees on their own initiative. In the following year it appointed a part-time physician to advise the directors of the association concerning "sick benefit" claims and give service for minor ailments. About 1920 a dental clinic was established and in 1932 a preventive program, including health examinations and diagnostic tests, was initiated. Up to 1932 the association had provided for sick benefits only. In that year it added hospital benefits. The association has continued to operate until the present. Its medical department was purchased by the firm in 1945 and has been maintained by it since.

A pattern which later assumed great importance was set by the Northern Pacific Railway Beneficial Association. Founded by the employees in 1882, this organization grew steadily and developed a program of complete medical care financed by prepayments and operated on the basis of group practice.

Fraternal beneficiary societies.—The fraternal beneficiary societies were organizations "working under ritual, holding regular lodge or similar meetings." The use of rituals and the emphasis on sociability and education distinguished these societies from the mutual benefit associations. One of their purposes was fraternal assistance to living members in sickness and destitution, payment of benefits to living members for total physical disability, and payment of benefits at the death of members to the families, heirs, blood relatives, or dependents. Insurance was an afterthought. Once it was introduced, it gained ground rapidly and soon became known as "fraternal insurance."

The godfather of such societies was the Ancient Order of United Workmen, founded in 1868, which was instrumental in organizing the National Fraternal Congress in Washington in 1896. There sixteen societies were represented and these had a membership of 535,000 carrying insurance protection of about $1,200,000,000.[4] Their annual expenditures for assistance to their members were substantial, as the reports showed, and this very fact disproved the notion that "sounding brass or a tinkling cymbal" was all they had to offer. The provisions for the sick were essentially remedial, and the practices followed in applying the insurance principle soon were attacked as unsound. As one critic remarked, "insurance" which does not protect is no insurance at all. In the course of development, life insurance and disability insurance came to occupy a dominant place. Provisions for medical care were an adjunct. Many societies began to employ "lodge doctors," who had to attend the members for a stipulated sum per member or a fixed salary, and some also used their resources for the construction, equipment, and maintenance of hospitals, primarily tuberculosis sanatoria.

An organization with all the features of mutual benefit associations and some characteristics of fraternal beneficiary societies is the Workmen's Benefit Fund of the United States, now an association with some 50,000 members and numerous branches in many parts of the country. It evolved out of a fraternal benefit society organized in 1884 and originally operated only in the vicinity of New York. In the early stage the object of the society, as stated in the constitution of 1890, was "to secure proper support to its members in case they are disabled from work by sickness, and to contribute towards the funeral expenses in case of their death." As time went on, other provisions, including periodic health examinations and care of the sick, were added. In New York City, for instance, provision is made for complete service by specialists and general practitioners, hospitalization, and convalescent care in a society-owned convalescent home for members discharged from the hospital.

Commercial insurance companies.—On May 1, 1847, a

young newspaper editor in Brooklyn applied for a life insurance policy in the sum of $2,500. A few days later he passed the physical examination given by the company physician, having been found "healthy, risk good." The applicant was accepted as a policyholder and signed the papers as Walter Whitman, Junior. He is better known as Walt Whitman.[5] The "Dreamer of the Great American Dream" who displayed so much foresight could not have taken out a life insurance policy a few years earlier because it was only in the early forties of the nineteenth century that commercial health insurance was first written in the United States. In 1850, limited coverage of wage loss due to accident was added to the health contracts of some companies, and in the sixties more extended coverage of such risks was offered. At the end of the nineties, payment of weekly indemnity for disability resulting from specified diseases was introduced, and by 1910 compensation for disability from all but a few diseases had become common practice.[6] "The period from 1850 to 1900 was one of experimentation for insurance underwriters in general. Of the unstable quality which characterized the business, health insurance was no more guilty than life insurance."[7] This fact is of more than historical interest. Other organizations entering the field of health insurance later paid little attention to the lessons learned by commercial companies before, repeated many of the early errors, and floundered expensively.

Industrial companies.—As industry expanded and the maintenance of a "healthy and vigorous labor force" became a crucial issue, more and more companies took steps to provide their employees with medical service and protection against the economic risks of disability and death. The lumber, coal mining, and metal mining industries and the railroad companies were most active in the field, and other industries followed suit. In most cases the employees had to contribute to the cost through a group prepayment plan, such as an employees' mutual benefit association. A typical example is the

Homestake Mining Company in the Black Hills district of South Dakota, which established a medical service in the seventies and had it financed by employee prepayments until 1910.[8]

Labor unions.—Toward the end of the nineteenth century, labor unions began to use revenues from general union dues or special contributions to provide their members with compensation in the event of death, dismemberment, and disability. These types of benefits continued to be developed while medical care insurance was largely ignored. However, some unions began to help their members by paying from their general funds toward the cost of physicians' service and of care in tuberculosis sanatoria and general hospitals. A few extended this policy to visiting nurse service and procurement of drugs and eyeglasses. An exceptional policy was adopted by the International Ladies' Garment Workers' Union. Several locals of this union banded together in 1913 to finance a clinic in the city of New York. Out of this primitive institution developed the present Union Health Center. Originally examination of candidates for membership in the locals and medical examination of the members claiming sick benefits were the chief functions of the institution, but beginning in 1930 diagnostic and treatment services and health education were added and extended. With the inclusion of provisions for a health and welfare fund in collective bargaining agreements, the Health Center came to play an increasingly important role in furnishing prepaid medical service to the union members.[9] The union also established health centers in Philadelphia and Fall River.

Distinctive features of the first phase.—The first phase of the development of voluntary medical care insurance extended into the second decade of the twentieth century. It was characterized by the introduction of certain practices which later came into wide use and by the development of certain patterns which led to bitter controversies.

Trends of Development 41

With very few exceptions the nonprofit organizations limited their activities to local communities, admitted primarily persons belonging to certain socioeconomic or occupational groups, and, directly or indirectly, required preliminary medical examination of applicants. The industrial plans usually accepted employees only. The method of payroll deduction was increasingly used to collect prepayments from employed persons. Commercial insurance policies were written on the basis of individual insurance and sold wherever the companies had agents. All organizations placed the emphasis on payment of cash benefits. Compensation was provided upon the occurrence of death, dismemberment, and disability resulting from disease and accident, although there were considerable variations in the scope of provisions.

Medical care insurance played a secondary role in the programs of all nonprofit associations except those in industry and was not written at all by commercial companies. Such medical care as was provided was often far from adequate in quality and quantity. The institutions of the "lodge doctor," the "company doctor," and the "camp physician," whatever their merits may have been in certain communities at the time, came in for denunciation in many parts of the country. The plan members complained about superficial and hasty service. The physicians felt exploited because their remuneration turned out to be far too low in proportion to the amount of service demanded. The medical profession resented the widespread policy of awarding contracts to the lowest bidder, registered strong opposition to the system of "contract practice" as it had developed, and set out to scrutinize agreements between physicians and organizations, such as industrial companies or consumer groups, as to unethical features.

REDISCOVERY AND EXPANSION

Voluntary medical care insurance entered the second phase of its evolution in the late twenties, expanded markedly in the thirties, and grew rapidly in the forties. The movement in the United States took a course similar in most respects to that followed by voluntary plans in European countries in the second half of the nineteenth century and the first two decades of the twentieth century.

The growth of medical care insurance in the United States was stimulated by the recognition of both the unmet needs in the field of health service and the necessity of budgeting for medical care.[10] Wide public interest was aroused by the studies of the Committee on the Costs of Medical Care [11] and of the United States Public Health Service.[12] The need for organized health programs was forcefully driven home by the severe economic crisis during the thirties. Recommendations for action by voluntary effort multiplied. It was the introduction of countless health service bills in Congress and state legislatures that, more than any other factor in the late thirties and early forties, spurred voluntary agencies "to do something about medical care."

The organizations which had long been interested in voluntary insurance plans extended their activities, improved their provisions, and grew in membership. Only the old-type fraternal benefit societies lost in relative importance, although some of them assumed considerable responsibility for the provision of hospital care, primarily in tuberculosis sanatoria.

Employees' mutual benefit associations.—After 1910, employees' mutual benefit associations increased in membership as well as number. By 1930, they had found a place for themselves in many industrial and mercantile concerns.[13] They were known to cover more than 600,000 workers in 306 plants, of which 158 had employee-managed associations, 28 had employer-managed associations, and 120 had organizations managed by employers and employees jointly.[14] A survey conducted in 1938 showed that in 248 companies employing 844,459 persons, 642,806 or 76.1 per cent were members of employees' mutual benefit associations.[15] By 1940, such organizations were in operation in 796 or 39 per cent of 2,064 plants returning information to the National Association of Manufacturers.[16] Approximately one half were financially aided by the employers. The large majority used the method of payroll deduction for the collection of dues.

The functions of the employees' mutual benefit associations had changed considerably since 1920. Death benefits had been increasingly discontinued because of the growth of group insurance sold by commercial insurance companies, although at the end of the thirties the majority of the associations still made such provisions. Disability benefits had been increased in amount. Hospital benefits had been included by a number of associations, although at the end of the thirties the majority of all associations did not provide for any type of medical care. The prevailing policy was to indemnify the members for part of the cost of specified care received. Service plans providing for a variety of essential services had been developed by a few associations only, such as the Allis-Chalmers Mutual Aid Society in West Allis, Wisconsin; the Consolidated Edison Employees' Mutual Aid Society, New York; the Stanocola Employees' Medical and Hospital Association in Baton Rouge, Louisiana; and the Union Oil Company of California Employees' Benefit Plan.

Commercial insurance companies.—In 1911 commercial insurance companies had introduced group insurance, defined as "an attempt by insurers to insure a number of individuals forming a group under a simple blanket policy at reduced rates." In the twenties they proceeded to write disability insurance covering sickness and nonoccupational accident in addition to loss of life, permanent disability, and temporary disability caused by occupational accident and disease. In the thirties they added "hospitalization indemnity," "surgical indemnity," and "medical indemnity" insurance covering nonoccupational illness and injury.

Industrial companies.—More and more companies in many

types of industry took steps to develop "health insurance" plans for their employees. Some started medical care plans as a part of a general welfare program designed to win employee loyalty and discourage union organization.[17] Others were motivated by the desire to safeguard the health of their employees and give them a sense of security, to reduce absenteeism due to illness, to attain most profitable production, and—last but not least—to improve labor-management relations. Their practices varied greatly, however. After 1920 an increasing number of corporations had their programs underwritten by commercial insurance companies. The master policies usually provided for "group health and accident insurance," covering disability due to sickness and nonoccupational accident, and for other types, such as life, accidental death, and dismemberment insurance. Since the late thirties, indemnification for hospital bills, physicians' bills, or both has been added more frequently. In 1938, the cost of group health and accident insurance was paid by the employees in 27 per cent of 144 companies studied, by employers in 7 per cent, and by both jointly in 66 per cent.[18]

A second and much smaller group of industrial companies followed an entirely different course. They initiated company-administered employees' mutual benefit associations or encouraged the establishment of such associations by the employees, retaining a varying degree of administrative control. A pertinent example is the Ansco Mutual Benefit Association of Binghamton, New York, organized in 1929 at two divisions of the General Aniline and Film Corporation. In some instances, administrative responsibility was transferred from the company to a board of directors elected by the plan members. Such a policy was adopted by the Union Oil Company of California, whose employees' benefit plan from its inception in 1915 until 1930 had been administered entirely by the company officials, and since that time has been managed by a board of six administrators representing the member-employees. In

1938, approximately half of the companies studied by the National Conference Board exercised some supervision over the associations, usually by appointing a management representative as one of the officers.[19] A few companies made it a condition of employment for applicants to join the association, but the great majority refrained from using compulsion. Many paid regular contributions toward the cost of the program or assisted the associations by furnishing administrative personnel, or did both. Examples are the Southern Pacific Company, San Francisco, California, and the General Aniline and Film Corporation, Binghamton, New York. Some companies also advanced funds or paid subsidies for the construction and equipment of necessary facilities. A pertinent example is the Standard Oil Company of Louisiana, Baton Rouge, Louisiana, which assisted the employee association in meeting the construction cost of a clinic building. A few industrial corporations, such as the Tennessee Coal, Iron and Railroad Company in Fairfield, Alabama, built all hospital and clinic facilities out of their own resources, financed the service for nonoccupational sickness and injury through a prepayment plan and for compensable conditions out of company funds, and took full administrative responsibility for their medical care programs. The extension of an industrial prepayment plan to all residents of the community was made possible in Roanoke Rapids, North Carolina, by the cooperative action of several industrial corporations.[20]

In recent years many employers have taken over part or all of the prepayments for employees enrolling in community-wide prepayment organizations such as Blue Cross or Blue Shield plans. It was the war emergency that spurred such practices. Both management and labor were anxious to provide the workers with tangible benefits in lieu of wage increases or in addition to a limited increase at a time when the wages were stabilized. Later this policy was continued not as a substitute for higher wages but as an added benefit for the common good and greatly extended under union-management agreements. Employer participation is facilitated by the fact that payments made by a company to a nonprofit health association on behalf of its employees are deductible as ordinary and necessary business expenses for Federal Income Tax purposes (Section 23a of the Internal Revenue Code).

A few industrial companies use exclusively resources of their own to pay for both capital expenditures and operating costs of medical care programs. In these cases neither the employees nor their eligible family dependents contribute to the maintenance of the services. Outstanding examples of such company-financed medical care programs are the Homestake Mining Company in the Black Hills district of South Dakota, which adopted this policy in 1910; the Endicott Johnson Corporation, Johnson City, New York, which organized its service in 1919; and the American Cast Iron Pipe Company, Birmingham, Alabama, which established its program in 1923.

Side by side with companies genuinely interested in the development of medical care for workers, there were others which believed in the old system of contract practice and kept it alive despite all changes that had taken place since the nineteenth century. They made a contract with one physician to furnish all medical care, raised the funds for it by deductions from the workers' pay—the "checkoff system," turned the money so received over to the physician, and left it to him to hire assistants on salary and pocket the profits. Some companies in the coal mining industry established a particularly unsavory record.[21]

Labor unions.—The labor unions accepted both medical care insurance and disability insurance as part and parcel of their program for the welfare of union members. By the end of the twenties, sixty-three unions of nationwide scope paid death benefits, fourteen paid permanent disability benefits, twelve paid sickness benefits, ranging from $4 to $10 per week for a period of seven to sixteen weeks, and twenty had some form of insurance,[22] but only a few provided for medical care insurance.[23] The picture changed radically after 1942. Since that time the unions have demanded and increasingly obtained the inclusion of employer-supported "health insurance" in collective bargaining agreements. The underlying concept is well expressed in one of these contracts as follows: "The company and the union recognize that the health of the employees is essential to the welfare of not only the workers but the industry as well." Early in 1947 approximately 1,250,000 employees were covered by health benefit plans negotiated by employers and unions; more than nine tenths were in the clothing, textiles, and coal mining industries.[24]

Some of these plans are administered solely by the union, others jointly by the union and the employer, and still others by commercial insurance companies. Three developments deserve special mention.

In 1945, the Joint Council of the Retail, Wholesale, and Department Store Union, CIO, made an agreement with a number of companies in St. Louis, Missouri. The companies pay the full contributions on behalf of their employees, and the medical services are rendered by a group-practice organization, the Labor Health Institute, which operates under the auspices of the union.

On May 29, 1946, the National Bituminous Wage Agreement was concluded between the Coal Mines Administrator and the United Mine Workers, AF of L. It covers approximately 450,000 miners in 3,000 mines in 23 states and contains provisions for the creation of a "medical and hospital fund" through payroll deductions and its administration by trustees appointed by the president of the union.[25]

On May 4, 1947, the first agreement with a basic steel producer calling for a company-financed health and welfare program was signed between the Allegheny Ludlum Steel Corporation and the United Steel Workers of America, CIO.

New organizations.—In the last three decades numerous

new organizations have assumed responsibility for health service plans based on the principle of insurance. In historical order of sequence they include institutions of higher learning, single hospitals, groups of physicians in private practice working together in the form of copartnerships, consumer cooperatives outside industry, county medical societies, community-sponsored nonprofit corporations for hospital service (Blue Cross plans), governmental agencies, state medical societies organizing nonprofit prepayment plans for physicians' service, and community-sponsored corporations providing for general programs of medical care. Details will be presented in the pertinent sections of Chapters Four to Eight.

Enabling legislation.—Establishment and operation of commercial insurance companies and of certain nonprofit organizations, such as fraternal beneficiary societies and mutual benefit associations, had long been regulated by law. The organization and maintenance of company-sponsored medical care programs for the employees of industrial and mercantile concerns rested on clear legal foundations, as the courts had confirmed the right of business concerns to take such action as part of the powers specifically granted in their certificates of incorporation. The right to organize and operate general nonprofit prepayment plans for hospitalization, professional services, or both was not beyond any doubt.

To clarify the situation, enabling acts for the formation of nonprofit hospital service plans and, in a later stage, of nonprofit physicians' service plans have been adopted by one state after another since the middle thirties. By the fall of 1946, thirty-six states had passed laws regarding nonprofit hospital service plans, and twenty-nine states had enacted laws dealing with medical service plans.[26]

The distinctive features of such legislation are the recognition of the right to organize nonprofit prepayment plans for hospital service, physicians' service, or both and the differentiation of such plans from organizations which offer a contract of insurance indemnifying policyholders for a monetary loss after its occurrence. As a general rule the commissioner of insurance is given considerable authority to regulate and supervise these plans. He has "the power to accept or reject the articles of incorporation and the application for license to operate and approve or disapprove the premium rates charged subscribers and the rates of payments to participating hospitals and physicians. After the plan has been in operation for a period, the commissioner is authorized to examine its affairs when he thinks necessary, scrutinize costs of administration, and rule on its solvency and ability to meet its obligations. Finally, the commissioner has the power to start proceedings against the corporation if he is of the opinion that it is not operating within the law and is hazardous to the public welfare." [27]

Distinctive features of the second phase.—The development since the twenties, haphazard and multiform as it was, differed strikingly from the earlier one both in kind and degree. Organization of medical care insurance came to receive primary attention, although disability insurance continued to be extended and improved.

The stock and mutual insurance companies concentrated on the sale of group insurance policies which usually did not require the applicants to pass a physical examination and thus were available to persons unable to obtain individual policies. Their scope of activities was greatly expanded with the inclusion of health benefits in collective bargaining agreements between management and labor—one of the most significant recent developments.

Nonprofit prepayment plans, varying in type and scope, were established in many parts of the country and increasingly on a state-wide basis. Enabling laws were passed by the majority of all states, in some instances with a definite tendency to create a monopoly for plans sponsored by the medical profession.

The prevailing policy was to organize separate plans for hospitalization and professional services and to provide for protection against the risks of "catastrophic illness" by offering first hospital service and later selected professional services, primarily surgical service in the hospital. More inclusive service was provided only by a few medical society plans, most of the group practice organizations, and many industrial programs.

Most plans emphasized family coverage rather than enrollment of breadwinners only and made more or less formal agreements with physicians in private practice and with hospitals regardless of ownership. The idea of cooperative ownership of the essential facilities, such as hospitals and clinics, gained ground, especially in industrial plants and rural areas. Organization of professional services on the basis of group practice made slow but definite progress in some parts of the country.

The service principle was adopted and maintained by important organizations, such as the Blue Cross plans, the group practice prepayment plans, and some of the individual practice plans sponsored by medical societies, but was rejected from the outset or abandoned in favor of the indemnity principle by many medical society plans.

The total number of persons enrolled in nonprofit prepayment plans of various types grew rapidly and came to exceed that of persons subscribing to plans operated for profit. Dual administration of nonprofit organizations became the prevailing policy, with one plan in charge of hospital service and another one administering physicians' service. Unified administration of more or less complete programs of medical care was the rule only in a relatively small number of nonprofit prepayment organizations, chiefly group practice and industrial plans. The principle of democratic control was determinedly applied by very few organizations, mainly the cooperatives within and outside industry and some of the community-sponsored plans. In this respect the development in the United States differed from that in European countries, which generally had placed the emphasis on full representation of the insured on the administrative bodies.

The motives guiding the development in the second phase were manifold. To paraphrase a statement made by Michael M. Davis, there were people who believed in and desired the extension of voluntary medical care insurance as a service to the public and a benefit to the health professions and hospitals. There were others whose motive was the hope of forestalling a compulsory system. In between were many who had thought little about these matters but who were willing to go along.[28]

CLASSIFICATION AND MEMBERSHIP OF PLANS

The medical care insurance plans now in operation are diverse in form of organization; auspices; type, scope, amount, and period of benefits; eligibility requirements; organization of professional services; method of payment for professional and hospital services; cost to subscribers; and administrative organization. At first glance the picture seems to be like a mosaic without any design. Closer study, however, reveals that there are definite patterns.

The existing organizations may be classified in various ways. They may be divided into nonprofit plans and plans operated for profit. They may be grouped according to the type of administrative control, such as control by medical societies, consumer cooperatives, private groups of physicians, or community organizations, or according to the socioeconomic groups covered by distinguishing industrial and rural plans. Useful as this approach may be, it does not bring out the very facts that determine the ultimate value of a plan applying the principle of insurance.

If the classification is to serve the measurement and appraisal of medical care insurance plans, it must take into account the basic policies followed in providing for benefits. Applying this principle, one may classify the existing plans in two broad categories, one comprising cash indemnity plans and the other one service plans. Each category may be subdivided according to the type of care provided, for example, hospitalization, physicians' service, or professional as well as hospital service. Organizations furnishing professional services may be grouped according to the pattern chosen for practice, such as individual and group practice. In each subdivision, nonprofit plans must be distinguished from plans operated for profit. The following is a systematic classification of medical care insurance plans.

A. Cash Indemnity Plans

1. Plans indemnifying for hospital expenses only
2. Plans indemnifying for professional expenses only
    (1) surgical expense indemnity plans
    (2) medical (nonsurgical) expense indemnity plans
    (3) plans indemnifying for surgical and nonsurgical expenses
3. Plans indemnifying for hospital and professional expenses

B. Service Plans

1. Plans providing for hospitalization only
    (1) free choice plans, organized to provide service by a number of participating hospitals
    (2) single hospital plans, organized to provide service by one hospital
2. Plans providing for physicians' service only
    (1) individual practice plans
    (2) group practice plans
3. Plans providing for hospitalization and professional services
    (1) individual practice plans
    (2) group practice plans

Accurate information on the total number of persons covered by medical care insurance plans is lacking. There are

Trends of Development 53

complete and reliable data on the number of participants in Blue Cross plans and fairly dependable figures on the enrollment in plans sponsored by medical societies and in a number of industrial, rural, and group-practice organizations.

All evidence points to the conclusion that the large majority of subscribers to medical society plans also are enrolled in Blue Cross plans, that many members of hospital service plans also hold commercial policies covering surgical expenses, and that most of the persons covered by commercial hospital insurance also are insured against the cost of surgical care. To add up the enrollment figures for all types of nonprofit plans or of commercial as well as nonprofit plans in order to determine the extent of insurance protection would be like adding up the passengers in automobiles, rather than the cars, in order to find out the amount of traffic going over a bridge. Moreover, some reports err on the side of overstatement by listing company-financed industrial programs and tax-supported plans that do not apply the basic principles of insurance and by including persons accepted on the basis of the fee-for-service system. For what they are worth the data are given here as published or furnished by the national organizations concerned.

Following up its first study in 1943, the Social Security Administration in 1945 supplied information on 229 prepayment medical care organizations with 4,975,850 members. They included 115 industrial plans with 1,512,074 persons; 53 medical society plans (including 22 in Washington and Oregon) with 2,594,356 persons; 21 private group clinic plans with 406,330 persons; 32 consumer-sponsored plans with 350,114 persons; and 8 governmental plans with 112,902 persons. The participants included 2,388,150 subscribers and 2,587,700 family dependents. Almost 44,000 physicians were giving care or had indicated their willingness to give care to the persons belonging to these organizations. Of these about 36,000 were "participating," nearly all being associated with medical society plans; 6,760 received salary for part-time service, about nine-tenths being with industrial plans; and 764 were employed on full-time salary, nearly two-thirds serving with industrial plans.[29] Substantial changes have taken place since.

At the end of 1946, there were 24,283,173 persons enrolled in hospital service plans approved by the American Hospital Association; about 5,000,000 persons enrolled in plans approved by the American Medical Association; about 10,500,000 persons carrying commercial group insurance policies for hospitalization indemnity, nearly 8,000,000 persons carrying commercial group policies for surgical indemnity, and about 600,000 persons carrying commercial group policies covering nonsurgical expenses.

It would require volumes to give a picture of the present situation in its complexity and prodigal variety. For practical purposes it appears sufficient to describe and evaluate the principal types of plans only, with due consideration to pattern of organization and administration and to actual experience.

THREE

Attitudes of National Voluntary Organizations

NEARLY all the national organizations representing the health professions, the voluntary hospitals, the farmers, labor, and industry and commerce have occasionally or repeatedly expressed their opinions on voluntary health insurance as such or on specific types of voluntary plans. The following summary gives excerpts of the most important statements officially adopted by national voluntary organizations since the thirties. It omits the many declarations dealing with the method of prepayment in general, such as the statement on "Nursing in Prepayment Plans" approved by the representative bodies of the American Nurses' Association and the National Organization for Public Health Nursing in 1946,[1] and excludes recommendations favoring compulsory insurance without direct or indirect reference to the voluntary method.

AMERICAN MEDICAL ASSOCIATION

The American Medical Association has long been on record as endorsing "voluntary health insurance." In numerous official statements it has elaborated upon the application of this principle to the organization of physicians' service and hospitalization and its relation to the method of group practice.

Physicians' service.—In 1934, the House of Delegates of the American Medical Association adopted a set of principles, one of which may be interpreted as relating to insurance: "However the cost of medical service may be distributed, the immediate cost should be borne by the patient if able to pay at the time the service is rendered."[2] In 1935, this was changed to read as follows: "In whatever way the cost of medical service may be distributed, it should be paid for by the patient in accordance with his income status and in a manner that is mutually satisfactory." [3] Earlier in the same year specific reference to voluntary insurance had been made in a resolution expressing "encouragement to local medical organizations to establish plans for the provision of adequate medical service for all of the people, adjusted to present economic conditions, by voluntary budgeting to meet the costs of illness." [4]

In the second half of the thirties the American Medical Association showed much concern over the type of insurance that should be sanctioned. In June, 1938, the House of Delegates accepted a report urging that "the benefits shall be paid in cash directly to the individual member. Thus, the direct control of medical service may be avoided. Cash benefits only will not disturb or alter the relations of patients, physicians and hospitals." [5] In September, 1938, it adopted a resolution stating ". . . it is practicable to develop cash indemnity insurance plans to cover, in whole or in part, the costs of emergency or prolonged illness . . ." and reaffirming the "conviction that voluntary indemnity insurance may assist many income groups to finance their sickness costs without subsidy." [6]

The wisdom of giving unqualified support to the indemnity principle must have been questioned by many members of the Association, as subsequent pronouncements indicate. In 1942, the House of Delegates approved the "principle of medical service plans on a service basis when sponsored by a constituent state medical association or a component county medical society in accordance with the recommendations relative to medical service plans adopted by the House of Delegates." [7] In 1943, in response to demand for more positive action, the "Council on Medical Service and Public Relations" was created to serve as a clearinghouse of information on medical care plans and to assist in their development.

The "Constructive Program for Medical Care" of June 22,

1945, called for "the development in or extension to all localities of voluntary sickness insurance plans and provisions for the extension of these plans to the needy under the principles already established by the American Medical Association," [8] and a resolution passed by the House of Delegates on December 5, 1945, urged "nationwide organization of locally administered prepayment medical plans sponsored by medical societies." [9]

In a restatement of the program of December, 1945, the Board of Trustees of the American Medical Association on February 14, 1946 declared:

A program for medical care within the American system of individual initiative and freedom of enterprise includes the establishment of . . . voluntary nonprofit prepayment plans for medical care (such as those developed by many state and county medical societies). The principles of such insurance contracts should be acceptable to the Council on Medical Service of the American Medical Association and to the authoritative bodies of state medical associations. The evolution of voluntary prepayment insurance against the costs of sickness admits also the utilization of private sickness insurance plans which comply with state regulatory statutes and meet the standards of the Council on Medical Service of the American Medical Association.[10]

Subsequently, preliminary "standards of acceptance for medical care plans" were issued. The requirements include approval of plans by the state medical association or the county medical society in whose area the plan operates; responsibility of the medical profession for the medical services included in the benefits; free choice of physician; maintenance of the patient-physician relationship; and a number of other points relating to organization and operation. The benefits of approved plans "may be in terms of cash indemnity or service units." [11] To carry out the many administrative tasks a nonprofit organization, Associated Medical Care Plans, was created. Its functions are to "promote the establishment and operation of such non-profit, voluntary medical care plans . . . as will adequately meet the health needs of the public and will preserve and advance scientific medicine . . ." Its bylaws call for compilation of statistics and distribution of financial and service data to member-plans, public education on the scope and significance of the prepayment movement, and encouragement of reciprocity among plans to facilitate enrollment of large, nationwide groups.

Hospital service.—The Judicial Council of the American Medical Association in 1926 warned against hospitalization plans organized "for the purpose of soliciting patients" [12] and in 1931 added economic considerations to the ethical argument by stating: "Within the last year, some community hospitals have announced their intention to provide medical, surgical and hospital service to families on a flat rate basis . . . In the cases presented to it, the Judicial Council has advised against the adoption of such plans by community hospitals because it is believed that they are not economically sound, in that they may be unfavorably affected by conditions entirely beyond control under which contracts cannot be fulfilled." [13] In 1933, the report of the officers of the American Medical Association declared that "group hospitalization represents a phase of contract practice which is comparatively new" and that the situation demanded "the immediate and serious consideration of the entire medical profession." [14] In 1935, the Association warned that "if hospitals are permitted to include medical services in their contracts for hospital care, the avenue is opened and the precedent set for the practice of medicine by hospitals." [15]

Faced with the fact that nonprofit hospital service plans were increasing in number and membership and spreading to many parts of the country, the American Medical Association in 1937 decided to formulate certain principles for the future development of hospitalization insurance, repeating its conviction that medical service should not be included in hospital service contracts.[16] In 1938, it passed a resolution approving "the principle of hospital service insurance which is being widely adopted throughout the country. It is susceptible of great expansion along sound lines, and your committee particularly recommends it as a community project. Experience in the operation of hospital service insurance or group hospitalization plans has demonstrated that these plans should confine themselves to provision of hospital facilities and should not include any type of medical care." [17]

This stand was reaffirmed in several subsequent pronouncements which, however, did not contain the term "hospital service insurance." The "Constructive Program for Medical Care," adopted on June 22, 1945, included a recommendation for "increased hospitalization insurance on a voluntary basis," [18] and the "National Health Program" of February 14, 1946, called for the establishment of "voluntary nonprofit prepayment plans for the costs of hospitalization (such as the Blue Cross plans). . . ." [19] The verbiage of these statements indicates continued adherence to the policy of separating hospitalization and physicians' service under insurance programs.

Group practice.—The appearance of group practice organizations was greeted by the medical profession with mixed feelings. Their potential value to the improvement and extension of medical care was realized but their impact on the practitioners in individual practice was dreaded. The bone of contention was not the principle of group practice but the method of paying for such service. The dispute arose when the physicians on the staff of a group clinic made an agreement with a third party to accept payment for their services on a basis other than the traditional fee-for-service system. It was the combination of group practice and group prepayment that stirred up bitter controversies.

As early as 1912 the Code of Ethics had branded as unethical "an agreement between a physician or a group of physicians, as principals or agents, and a corporation, organization . . . or individual, to furnish . . . medical services to a group or class of individuals on the basis of a fee schedule, or for a salary or a fixed rate per capita." [20] In 1926, the Judicial Council of the American Medical Association condemned "the solicitation of patients whether by individual physicians, by groups, by institutions, or by organizations of physicians" and specifically referred to "health or hospital associations," which were declared "distinctly unethical" if organized for the purpose of soliciting patients. Physicians were warned "to guard themselves against being connected with such organizations." [21] It was on ethical grounds that the national organization of the medical profession objected to group practice paid for through a prepayment plan. In 1934, the American Medical Association defined the specific "features or conditions" making a contract unethical and embodied its views in an amendment to its "Principles of Medical Ethics" as follows:

Contract practice *per se* is not unethical. However, certain features or conditions if present make a contract unethical, among which are: 1. When there is solicitation of patients, directly or indirectly. 2. When there is underbidding to secure the contract. 3. When the compensation is inadequate to assure good medical service. 4. When there is interference with reasonable competition in a community. 5. When free choice of a physician is prevented. 6. When the conditions of employment make it impossible to render adequate service to the patients. 7. When the contract because of any of the provisions or practical results is contrary to sound public policy . . .

The decision as to its [contract practice] ethical or unethical nature must be based on the ultimate effect for good or ill on the people as a whole.[22]

The ethical argument was again stressed in 1940 when the Bureau of Medical Economics reported to the House of Delegates as follows:

Although the American Medical Association and its constituent societies have been charged with opposition to group practice, a search of the Proceedings of the House of Delegates of the American Medical Association for thirty-two years failed to show any action that indicated the slightest hostility to the formation of ethical and capable medical groups. The extent of the participation of group members as officials of the national and state organizations would indicate a complete absence of any such hostility.[23]

Ethics has always been a flexible notion and concepts have changed with developments. There are physicians who believe that any method of organizing medical care is ethical if it serves the ultimate good of the people at large and that group practice is such a method. Actually many of the physicians who in the thirties assumed the leadership in organizing group practice prepayment plans were punished for their action. They were expelled from their medical society and consequently lost the hospital privilege, teaching appointments, opportunity for consultation, the right to accreditation by specialty boards, and the possibility of taking out malpractice insurance policies or obtaining malpractice defense without great cost. Their hospitals were removed from the list of hospitals registered by the American Medical Association.[24]

The problem of group practice aroused great public interest, and one of the books on it received much attention.[25] The controversy was settled in 1943 by a unanimous ruling of the Supreme Court against the American Medical Association in the test case of the Group Health Association of Washington, D.C. The decision pointed out that the medical societies had combined and conspired to prevent the successful operation of this organization by taking the following steps: "(1) to impose restraints on physicians affiliated with Group Health by threat of expulsion or actual expulsion from the societies; (2) to deny them the essential professional contacts with other physicians, and (3) to use coercive power of the societies to deprive them of hospital facilities for their patients." [26]

AMERICAN DENTAL ASSOCIATION

In 1938, the House of Delegates of the American Dental Association adopted a statement of eight principles which in their opinion constituted the basis of any effective program of dental care. Thus constructive recommendations were substituted for the earlier negative approach of merely condemning "compulsory health insurance." In this pronouncement no reference was made to the method of paying for dental service. However, the same meeting accepted a report of a special committee which rejected a "compulsory health insurance system" and approved "voluntary budget plans under professional control." [27] Soon after, a special committee, known as the American Dental Association National Health Program Committee, was appointed by the Board of Trustees. It offered the opinion that "any service short of complete dental care would not be satisfactory and that it would be financially impossible for any compulsory health insurance system to furnish complete dental care to insured persons." [28] In 1941, a pamphlet issued by this committee briefly discussed various types of prepayment plans and "group plans," implying although not specifically mentioning the voluntary approach.[29]

AMERICAN HOSPITAL ASSOCIATION

On February 13, 1933, the American Hospital Association endorsed "the basic principle of periodic payment for the purchase of hospital care." [30] Since that time it has actively participated in the development and improvement of nonprofit organizations operating hospital service plans (see Chapter Five) and, also, repeatedly stressed the need for extension of the insurance principle to medical service.

As early as 1938, the House of Delegates of the American Hospital Association announced that it was "prepared to approve periodic payment plans for hospital care and medical service in hospitals," invited the medical profession to cooperate in the formulation of more acceptable plans, and outlined a set of principles.[31] In 1939, it reaffirmed "the importance and the desirability of applying the principle of voluntary insurance to both hospital and medical service for hospitalized cases among low income groups" and renewed its invitation to the American Medical Association to participate in the establishment of such plans.[32] In 1942 it adopted "Principles for Provision of Hospital Care," one of which called for "cooperation in the development in each community of nonprofit plans for medical service for hospital cases, sponsored by the medical profession . . ." [33]

ORGANIZATIONS OF FARMERS

Since the middle thirties the national organizations of farmers have intensified their efforts to improve the health conditions in rural areas. They have been and continue to be divided in their opinions about voluntary health insurance.

The National Grange, the oldest of the national organizations, in general has taken the position that voluntary plans are preferable to "compulsory government insurance." In its first positive statement on voluntary plans in 1940 it declared ". . . we look with favor on various voluntary plans for group medical care that are now in operation" and registered opposition to compulsory plans.[34] In 1944, it accepted a committee report recommending "that all Granges be urged actively to initiate or assist with the participation in groups for group hospital benefits for Grange members, such as Blue Cross Insurance, and other voluntary associations." [35] In 1945, the following resolution was adopted: "That because of the uneven and unpredictable cost of illness, it is of prime importance that rural people should spread the risks and share the costs of sickness by developing a comprehensive form of prepayment plans for hospital bills and health insurance." Clearly realizing the economic barrier to the development of voluntary plans, the National Grange at the same time called for financial help by resolving: "That since many rural families and rural areas are too poor to support doctors and hospital services even with any form of health insurance, public or private funds be combined with insurance funds to equalize the ability of these families and these areas to secure and maintain needed health services." [36] The Legislative Program 1947, adopted at the 80th Annual Session of the National Grange in 1946, contained a section on "rural health" which favored "development of cooperative measures for the improvement of rural health," opposed "compulsory federal medicine," and urged the initiation of "a medical-cost prepayment system which will enable all people to secure modern medical care without undue burden." [37]

The American Farm Bureau Federation lately has taken about the same position as the National Grange. Although it declared its support of legislation in 1938, it went on record against bills introduced in Congress later and expressed interest in the development of voluntary plans. At the annual convention in 1946 its affiliate, the Associated Women of the Federation, passed a resolution favoring "voluntary prepayment plans that will encourage doctors to establish themselves in rural areas" and recommending "support of the prepayment plans for hospitals, surgical and medical services." [38]

The Farmers Educational and Cooperative Union of America, known as the "National Farmers Union," in 1937 adopted a resolution supporting "the principles of group medicine and hospitalization on a Co-Operative basis, with fixed prepayment provisions covering individuals and families." [39] In the following year it testified in favor of legislation and later consistently endorsed proposals calling for compulsory programs, although it did not rule out voluntary organization. At the annual convention in 1944 it accepted a general program "Conservation of Human Resources," which contained a recommendation concerning the improvement of rural health services. The proposed program should "supplement the medical care provisions of the social security program expanded along the lines proposed by the Wagner-Murray-Dingell Bill." [40]

LABOR UNIONS

The American Federation of Labor and the Congress of Industrial Organizations regard voluntary health insurance as a stop-gap and want it replaced by a system of compulsory insurance, while the twenty Standard Railway Labor Unions have not committed themselves officially.

The American Federation of Labor in 1938 stated its conviction that "only a compulsory way is practical," [41] in 1939 endorsed "the principle of compulsory health insurance" as recommended in legislation then pending,[42] and in subsequent years continued to urge federal legislation. Its stand on voluntary plans is indicated by the following statement made by the Executive Council in 1940: "We approve of voluntary cooperation in the medical service field to the limits of its effectiveness, but we believe a comprehensive national health program is essential for our Nation." [43]

The Congress of Industrial Organizations at its first Constitutional Convention in 1938 passed one resolution endorsing the national health program then proposed and another one on "health cooperatives" which said: "Participation in such schemes is no substitute for a national health program, but they do tend to accustom both physicians and patients to thinking in terms of distributing the cost of medical care among the entire community." [44] Similar opinions were expressed later. In 1939, the CIO reaffirmed its "support for the immediate adoption of a program for insurance for medical care on a Federal basis" and advised its members that "as a spur to the adoption of the foregoing program, wherever possible CIO unions assist in the formation of general medical cooperatives in their communities." [45] In 1941, it passed a resolution on "medical cooperatives and non-profit medical insurance" urging the members to insist on "labor participation in the control of any health insurance plans" recommended by the CIO unions to their membership.[46] In recent years the CIO like the AF of L has thrown the weight of its influence behind legislative proposals for compulsory plans.

The Railway Labor Executives' Association, an association of the chief executive officers of twenty standard railway labor organizations, in May, 1946, agreed on a "health and welfare program" containing the following paragraph:

Many employers in the several branches of the transportation industry maintain in one form or another health and welfare benefits. A number of the railroads operate medical services for their employes, but for the most part the employes pay for the maintenance of these services through regular payroll deductions. There are a few instances where these medical services are jointly administered and controlled by representatives of both management and labor union officials. Many employers make available to the employes group insurance through payment of premiums by payroll deductions. In some instances there are programs for relief of sick and distressed employes. There are some plans for home purchase loans. The labor organizations should promptly formulate and seek adoption of comprehensive programs for medical care, life insurance, and other necessary benefits to be furnished by the industry and under joint administration of labor and management representatives.[47]

The International Association of Machinists at its convention in 1945 adopted a resolution on "provision for hospitalization in agreements with managements or other employers," calling among other things for adequate representation on the administrative agencies in charge of hospital service plans and for opportunity to "sit in on the drawing up of agreements with management or other employers." [48]

INDUSTRY AND COMMERCE

The Chamber of Commerce and the National Association of Manufacturers have officially come out in favor of voluntary plans.

The Chamber of Commerce of the United States in 1944 adopted a general policy with respect to social security and in this connection declared: "Voluntary group effort to provide more adequate medical services for all the people is urged." [49]

The National Association of Manufacturers has long been on record as endorsing voluntary plans. To supplement this position its Board of Directors on May 24, 1946, adopted a statement that the National Association of Manufacturers

    a. Encourage and stimulate the development of voluntary prepaid medical and health programs.
    b. Provide members with information regarding the operation and benefits to be derived from voluntary prepaid medical and health programs.
    c. Give wide distribution of information regarding such programs as are already in operation.[50]

On February 28, 1947, the Board of Directors accepted a statement on the position of the National Association of Manufacturers with regard to employee benefit programs. This pronouncement begins with the following declaration: "The NAM believes that employee benefit programs, including health and welfare programs, available to employees on a voluntary basis, have in most cases proved to be important factors in sound industrial relations." [51]

FOUR

Cash Indemnity Plans

CASH indemnity plans are designed to assist participants in paying the costs actually incurred for medical care. They allow stipulated sums of money up to a certain maximum toward the insured's expenses for specified professional services, hospital care, or both. Prepayments are collected and reimbursement is made according to a definite schedule. Indemnities in the amounts and for the period set forth in the contract are paid to the insured upon written notice and verification of his claim, or direct payments are made to the attending physician upon approval of his bills by the administrative office of the organization. The benefits are not intended to fix the value of physicians' services or to relate to such values.

Policies containing such provisions have long been sold by commercial insurance companies. Nonprofit plans applying these principles have been developed sporadically in industry and more frequently by organizations endorsed by medical societies.

COMMERCIAL INSURANCE POLICIES

History and trends of development.—Commercial insurance companies have taken the leadership in organizing indemnification for specified professional and hospital expenses. In 1903, the first successful attempt was made to add indemnification for surgical bills to individual insurance policies. This step, significant as it was as a venture into a new field, did not find much response from the public. With the introduction of group insurance and the extension of such policies to include indemnity for certain medical care bills, the situation changed. Increasingly hospital expense indemnity insurance has been written since the thirties, surgical expense indemnity since the end of the thirties, and medical (nonsurgical) expense indemnity since the early forties. While group insurance policies came to play a steadily growing role in the insurance business, individual policies continued to be sold in substantial numbers.

It was the attitude of both management and labor that broadened the market for group insurance policies covering medical care expenses. Since the late thirties, more and more industrial corporations and business firms on their own accord have added hospitalization, surgical, and medical benefits to group insurance policies purchased from commercial insurance companies or have contributed toward the cost of such benefits by paying amounts ranging from one fourth to one half. They developed hospitalization insurance first and surgical indemnity later, beginning with coverage of the employees and proceeding to inclusion of family dependents. Already during the war and more frequently after its end, management accepted financial responsibility for such provisions under collective bargaining agreements with unions.

Cooperation with organizations of farmers recently offered a new opportunity for commercial insurance companies to extend their activities. An example is the agreement signed in 1946 between the California Farm Bureau Federation and three insurance companies in California. This contract covers hospitalization, surgical, and medical benefits and is handled by the Federation through its county bureaus and their farm centers.

The total number of persons covered by commercial policies insuring the expenses of specified types of medical care has grown continuously and substantially since the end of the thirties. This fact, however, cannot be substantiated accurately, as dependable figures are lacking. According to various estimates, some 300,000 persons were covered for hospital expenses and about 94,000 for surgical expenses in 1938;

about 2,550,000 persons for hospital expenses and about 1,575,000 for surgical expenses in 1940; and about 13,000,000 persons for hospital expenses, about 9,400,000 for surgical expenses, and less than 800,000 for nonsurgical expenses at the end of 1946. The great majority of these persons are insured under group insurance policies, and a relatively small proportion are carrying individual insurance policies. At the end of 1946, group hospital expense insurance covered approximately 5,800,000 employees and about 4,748,000 family dependents; group surgical expense insurance, about 5,392,000 employees and about 2,524,000 family dependents; and group medical expense insurance, about 490,000 employees and 125,000 family dependents.[1]

Eligibility requirements.—The organized plans underwritten by commercial carriers accept regularly employed persons enrolling in groups regardless of their income and without preliminary physical examination. Normally they require a minimum number of persons, such as twenty-five or fifty, and at least 75 per cent of the eligible employees to sign up and be insured. Age limits are uncommon. Eligibility begins after a specified period of employment which ranges from one to several months. The employee meeting this requirement must apply within a certain number of days of the date on which he first becomes eligible. The right to eligibility ends with termination of employment or upon retirement, although there are exceptions to this rule. Usually certain benefits are extended for a stipulated period if employment is discontinued due to disabling illness. Surgical benefits, for instance, are provided for three months in such cases.[2]

Not infrequently the wife of the employee and his unmarried children over three months but under eighteen years of age are eligible for specified benefits, chiefly hospital indemnity, under widely varying financial arrangements.

Individual policies offered to the general public normally are issued without prior medical examination to those applicants who state on a prescribed form that they themselves and all other persons whose names are listed on the application are in good health and have no disease or ailment which may require hospitalization or surgical operation. As a general rule they are available to persons below a certain age, such as sixty-five or seventy years, and may be taken out for dependent minors under eighteen years of age.

Type of illness covered.—The policies provide for benefits in the event of nonoccupational illness and accident. There are, however, many restrictions on the type of conditions for which reimbursement of charges can be claimed. Any disease or injury requiring hospitalization is covered under contracts indemnifying for the cost of hospital care. Only specified surgical conditions treated in the hospital are covered by policies providing for reimbursement of surgical expenses. Nonsurgical conditions entitle the holder of a "medical expense" policy to stipulated benefits that are usually allowed during the period of disability. Family contracts almost always include obstetrical care of the wife of the policyholder, subject to a waiting period of nine months or more.

Type and scope of benefits.—The basic types of benefits provided by the policies of commercial insurance companies are three: "hospital benefits," that is, payment toward the expenses of hospital care; "surgical benefits"—payment toward the cost of surgical and auxiliary services performed in the hospital; and "medical benefits"—payment toward the expenses of treatment for nonsurgical conditions in the hospital only or in the home and office as well as in the hospital. The first two types of benefits are common, hospital benefits being provided most frequently, and the third type is in the process of development.

As a general rule, limitations are imposed on the amounts of indemnification for specified types of expenses, the number of reimbursable services, the period of payment per case of illness or per contract year, and the total sum allowed during a period of disability or in the course of a year. The maximum amounts obtainable are set forth in special schedules. Occasionally they are graded according to the size of the premium paid. Policies covering benefits for nonsurgical conditions, in particular those including home and office calls, often contain a "deductible clause" excluding from reimbursement the expenses for a certain number of visits, such as the first two or three in any illness, or limiting claims to obligations incurred after the first three days of illness.

A typical commercial policy for hospital, surgical, and medical benefits, as sold early in 1947, made the following provisions for the insured employees: reimbursement for hospital expenses at the rate of $4.00 to $5.00 per day of hospitalization up to seventy days during any one period of disability and up to fourteen days in case of pregnancy, including resulting childbirth or miscarriage; reimbursement for surgical expenses up to the amounts specified in a "schedule of operations" and not exceeding a total of $150 for all operations performed during any one period of disability; reimbursement for the expenses of treatment by a duly qualified physician of nonsurgical conditions at the rate of not more than $2.00 for an office or hospital visit and $3.00 for a home visit, with a limit of $150 for all visits for treatment during any period of disability or for all visits for treatment in any twelve consecutive months after the sixtieth birthday of the employee. Eligible family dependents are entitled to hospital benefits up to a sum equal to 31 times the amount applicable in the case of employees and to 50 per cent of the maximum payment on account of surgeons' fees. They are not covered for medical benefits.

Policies providing for hospital, surgical, and medical expense indemnification often are supplemental to others, such as group accident and sickness policies, and in these cases are written in the form of riders attached to a single policy issued to the employer. Inclusive plans for employed persons are in wide use. They combine accidental death and dismemberment benefits, weekly accident and sickness benefits, hospital expense benefits, surgical expense benefits, and medical expense benefits.

The group insurance plan negotiated between the American Woolen Company and the Textile Workers' Union of America, CIO, which is underwritten by a commercial insurance company, provides for (1) weekly accident and sickness benefits in case of disability due to noncompensable accident or sickness and in the event of disability due to pregnancy or complications therefrom; (2) benefits in case of accidental death, dismemberment and loss of sight; (3) medical expense benefits in case of disability, beginning with the first call for accidents and the fourth call for sickness, at the rate of $2.00 for office calls and $3.00 for home or hospital calls, with a maximum of three calls in any one week and fifty calls in any one continuous disability; (4) surgical expense benefits up to $150 according to the special schedule attached to the policy; (5) hospital expense benefits, including allowances up to $6.00 per day or a total of $186.00 for board and room, up to $300.00 for sera, oxygen, oxygen tent, face mask, and helium, and up to $60.00 for other hospital charges and physician's fees for anesthesia. In maternity cases the maximum reimbursement is $84.00 for board and room and $30.00 for other charges. The cost of all benefits for employees is borne by the company. Certain family dependents of employees may be included in the hospital insurance program upon payment by the employee of $1.14 per month for one dependent and $1.64 per month for two or more dependents.

Individual insurance policies are much like the group insurance policies in regard to the type of provisions and the extent of indemnification. Usually they pay the "actual, reasonable and necessary charges" up to a maximum per year, although often minor expenses, such as the first $25, are not reimbursable.

Professional and hospital services.—Commercial insurance companies underwriting medical care insurance policies do not make contractual agreements with physicians and hospitals to guarantee service to the policyholders. They merely collect and disburse funds for the payment of bills incurred by the policyholders.

Regardless of the type of their policy, the insured choose the physician and hospital they wish to have, obtain such services as they desire, pay for care at the fees charged by those who have rendered the service, submit their claims together with evidence of their financial obligations to the administrative agency designated in their contract, and upon verification of their claims receive from the insurance carrier or administrative agency cash reimbursement in the amount stipulated in the policy.

The attending physicians are free to charge the patient according to their own estimate of the value of their services and their understanding with the patient, and the hospitals bill him on the basis of the usual rates. If the amounts payable exceed the indemnification received by the policyholder, the difference must be paid by him.

Premium rates.—The monthly premium rates charged in 1946 under group insurance policies covering employees were approximately $0.45 to $0.70 for hospital benefits, depending on the extent of coverage, $0.40 for surgical benefits, and $0.75 to $0.85 for surgical and medical benefits as described on p. 72. They increase progressively with the rise of the proportion of women and nonwhite employees beyond 10 per cent, and they are higher in hazardous industries. The monthly rates for both employees and family dependents in 1946 were about $1.35 to $2.15 for hospital benefits only, about $1.50 for surgical benefits without obstetrical care, and about $2.00 for obstetrical as well as surgical benefits.

In many instances the employers bear part or all of the cost of the benefits for the insured employees in accordance with a collective bargaining agreement, and in some instances they also pay a substantial proportion of the premium for the family dependents.

The premium rates of individual insurance policies are usually slightly higher than those of group insurance. They are payable monthly, quarterly, semiannually, or annually and are relatively lowest if payment is made for a full year in advance.

Administration.—Responsibility for the direct administration of the benefits provided under commercial group insurance policies is vested in the employer only, a union only, or employer and union jointly. Under the system of joint administrative control, clearly defined powers, duties, and functions are assigned to a board of trustees, which usually includes an impartial public member as chairman and representatives of the employers and the union, and to a supervisory committee consisting of employer and union representatives, and the chairman of the board.[3]

Experience.—It is fair to assume that there is a substantial body of experience in regard to cash indemnity plans sold by private insurance companies. Unfortunately few data other than fiscal are presented in reports. What is most regrettable is the dearth of published statistics on such basic questions as the number, sex, and age of persons submitting claims for the various benefits, the type and number of services for which reimbursement has been claimed and received, the major causes of illness, the cost of the various types of benefits per eligible person and per case, and the expenditures for administration.

A sample study recently made in the textile industry analyzed the experience of approximately 200 persons who were covered by a union-management contract underwritten by a commercial insurance company. The findings showed a wide margin between the benefits obtained and the actual expenditures made by this group. The employees received hospital benefits in an amount equal to 60 per cent of their expenses for hospital care, and combined hospital and surgical benefits equal to an amount covering 32 per cent of all their expenditures for hospitalization and professional services. In the case of the family dependents, the reimbursement for hospitalization costs constituted 48 per cent of the actual expenditures for this type of care and 21 per cent of the total cost incurred for hospital service and medical attention.[4]

One point is beyond doubt. The commercial insurance companies, well versed in the actuarial problems as they are, know that ". . . the insurance industry will not be able to supply on any substantial scale the comprehensive insurance plans" desired by the advocates of voluntary action.[5] Precisely for this reason they have concentrated their efforts on the sale of reasonably priced contracts for strictly limited benefits.

Achievements.—By accepting applicants regardless of income, the commercial companies have avoided the creation of a "poor man's system" with all its disadvantages. By selling low-priced policies covering selected benefits, they have made some medical care insurance available to substantial numbers of people in many parts of the country, especially to industrial employees. The inclusion of a large variety of benefits in one master policy and the offer of company-wide or trade-wide contracts with identical benefits for all employees in similar occupations and income groups has proved to be attractive to both employers and unions, as many types of health and welfare benefits are included, the benefits are equal for all participants, and the agreement can be made with one insurance carrier instead of numerous organizations.

The persons covered by these policies obtain a certain degree of protection against the economic hazards resulting from nonoccupational disease and injury. They are benefited most if they need hospitalization and surgical care involving a total cost of less than about $200. The physicians and hospitals profit by the increased purchasing power of the patients as well as the wide scope of free choice.

Shortcomings.—The great majority of the persons covered by cash indemnity policies are employees of industrial and business firms and self-employed people in the middle and higher income brackets. The low-income groups outside industry have not been reached to any significant extent. The family dependents of insured persons often are eligible for partial indemnity only. Reimbursement is confined to selected types of bills; it is limited by ceilings on the number of reimbursable services and on the amounts of money allowed for each type of service and for a specified period of time. In cases of serious illness the indemnity meets only a small fraction of the total obligations of the sick. The larger his actual expenditures, the smaller the percentage received as reimbursement. In cases of minor nonsurgical illness the patient is expected to bear part of the cost. Preventive medicine is ignored as the sole emphasis is placed on treatment of sickness or injury. There are no safeguards against overcharges of physicians or against possible misuse of the indemnity by patients.

Designed to equalize the financial impact of illness, the commercial cash indemnity plans cannot contribute to the improvement of the quality of medical care. Without minimizing the importance of financial arrangements for the payment of a part of doctor and hospital bills, it must be stated that such plans afford only a partial answer to one segment of the total problem.

NONPROFIT PLANS IN INDUSTRY

At a small number of industrial plants, nonprofit employee associations have been founded for the purpose of indemnifying the members for specified expenses due to nonoccupational disease and injury. The principles adopted for the organization of benefits are similar to those followed by commercial companies, but details of procedure differ. The management of the plans is in the hands of the employee-members. The three plans described in this section have been chosen as representative of the various methods of organization and administration. All three cover professional and hospital expenses of employees, although to a varying extent, and two also indemnify family dependents of employees. One plan is compulsory.

The *Union Oil Company of California Employees' Benefit Plan* was established by the company in 1915 and for fifteen years administered by its officials. In 1930 a board of six employees, elected by mail ballot, was authorized to manage the organization.

The object of the plan, according to its rules and regulations, is "to provide for the payment, within the limits . . . set forth . . . , of medical, surgical and hospital expenses incurred by members in non-industrial illnesses and accidents. . . ."

Any employee who completes three months' continuous service or one year of accumulated service is required to become a member of the plan, effective the first day of the month following the completion of such service. However, eligibility is restricted to male employees under forty-nine years and six months and female employees under forty-four years and six months on the date of entering employment. Passing of a physical examination "to the satisfaction of the company" is a prerequisite for acceptance. All rights in the plan cease with termination of employment, retirement from the company, or change to part-time employment of less than three eight-hour days per week. A plan member receiving treatment under the plan at the time when membership is terminated is entitled to continued benefits for a period up to six months or an expenditure not exceeding $500, provided he remains under continuous care of a panel doctor. The members numbered

6,375 at the end of 1930, 7,924 at the end of 1940, and 6,883 in April, 1947.

The plan pays "for all reasonable medical, surgical and hospital services" for noncompensable illnesses or injuries except "any illness or disability caused by or resulting directly or indirectly from any abnormal or defective condition or ailment which originated prior to the member's date of eligibility," any condition due to a deflection of the nasal septum, flat feet, pyorrhea, venereal diseases, obstetrical attention, injuries acquired willfully or sustained while committing a felony, conditions due to intoxication or the use of drugs, optical refractions, dentistry, tonsillectomy (with qualifications), drugs and medicines other than those prescribed and used while a member is hospitalized, medical supplies not recommended and approved by the attending physician, sickroom supplies, and special nursing. The board of directors may authorize payments up to $50 for expenses incurred in determining whether or not a member is suffering from a condition, disease, or ailment which is listed under the exclusion rule or existed prior to the date of the employee's eligibility.

The maximum allowed to a member in any one illness or condition was $500 until recently but was raised to $750 in the fall of 1947. Payment is also made in the event of recurrence of the same illness upon the expiration of two years of uninterrupted recovery.

The member must report any illness to the plan to secure authorization of benefits and has the right to choose his own physician from the lists of selected physicians and surgeons appointed by the board of administrators. The participating physicians receive direct payment from the plan according to a regular fee schedule. The reports of the attending physicians are carefully scrutinized by the administration, with special emphasis on indications for specialist care. In such cases consultation of selected specialists or referral of the patient is suggested. In 1947, approximately 600 physicians, including specialists and general practitioners, were cooperating with the organization. Local hospitals are utilized for bed care and paid the prevailing rates for ward service.

The prepayments are deducted from the members' payroll. The monthly rate charged early in 1947 was $2.00. Increase to $3.00 is under consideration.

The organization is managed by a board of six administrators, elected by the plan members for three-year terms, and elected officers, all serving without compensation. The board of administrators is charged with the duty of hearing and determining controversies in regard to the benefits and obligations of members, reviewing quarterly the financial affairs of the plan and recommending to the company any necessary adjustments in the prepayment rates, providing for reports of services rendered to members, and submitting annual reports.

The company bears the cost of administration of the plan by furnishing office space and the necessary administrative personnel, acting as a depositary for all contributions, making the disbursements, and providing for incidentals.

The *Columbia Employees' Hospitalization Plan* at Torrance, California, was incorporated in 1941 as a nonprofit organization and operates in accordance with the California State Insurance Code. Its purpose is to pay expenses incurred by the members due to noncompensable accident or illness.

The privilege of participation is extended to employees of the Columbia Steel Company of Torrance and their family dependents, including wife and children. There is no age or income limit. Neither is physical examination required. Eligibility for benefits begins ninety days after signing for and continuing membership. Six months of membership are necessary to qualify for benefits for chronic conditions and "for an illness or ailment not common to both sexes" in the case of female members. No payment is made for oral surgery, plastic surgery for cosmetic purposes, or vasectomies.

Cash Indemnity Plans

The benefits include allowances for both professional services and hospitalization. Indemnification for medical attendance and treatment is made for a total of sixty calls (home, office, or hospital) in any single illness or injury and for the fees of surgeons, assistant surgeons, and anesthetists in case of hospitalization. Unless the employee is disabled for at least two days, he must pay for the first two calls. The first call, however, is covered by the plan if minor surgery or first aid is required. Reimbursement of expenses for diagnostic X-ray and laboratory services to nonhospitalized members is limited to $80 in any single illness or injury. Payment for hospitalization is made at current ward rates for a period not exceeding ninety days in any one year or in any case of hospitalization. An additional sum up to $100 is allowed toward charges for use of the operating room, anesthesia, laboratory and X-ray services, drugs, and ambulance. The maximum indemnity available for any one illness or injury is $1,000.

The plan members have free choice of any licensed physician, surgeon, osteopathic physician or hospital in the area. Early in 1947 more than 700 physicians were cooperating. The fees allowed for the services of professional persons are set forth in a schedule specifying the maximum amounts of reimbursement for each type of service. Payment of specialists' bills is subject to prior authorization of such service by the claim committee of the plan. All approved claims are paid directly to the physicians or hospitals.

The monthly prepayment rates charged in 1947 were $3.00 for male and $3.50 for female plan members. Administrative responsibility is vested in a board of seventeen elected directors, six of whom constitute a "claim committee" in charge of approving allowances. The company does not participate in the management or operation of the plan. It assists the organization by furnishing telephone, mail service, and mimeograph work.

The *Spaulding Employees' Mutual Benefit Association*,

Binghamton, New York, was organized in 1930 by joint action of the company and the employees. Its object is "to assist members in case of sickness, accident or disability which may unfit them for their daily work."

Membership is open to employees and officers of the plant employed at least one month regardless of income and age, provided they are "in good health." Persons who file application for membership after the first month of employment must pass a physical examination. In addition, any member who is receiving benefits must submit to a physical examination by the "association physician" whenever required by the board of trustees. Family dependents of members, including the wife and children under eighteen years, are eligible for reimbursement of specified expenditures.

The benefits for employee-members apply to diseases and injuries not covered by the Workmen's Compensation law and include weekly sick benefits and indemnification of bills for professional and hospital services. Sick benefits are available for a period not exceeding ten weeks in any one year; they are not paid while members are hospitalized. Medical and hospital benefits are granted upon application to and authorization by the board of trustees. Allowances for medical care expenditures are made for the services of physicians, both general practitioners and specialists, in the home, office, and hospital, including one physical examination a year, major and minor operations, and treatment of eye, ear, nose, and throat diseases; dental care, including X-ray examinations and extractions up to an amount of $25 in any one year; diagnostic clinical laboratory and X-ray services; and general hospital care up to thirty days in any one year at the rate of $5.00 per day for ward service. Maternity care is excluded. The total amount paid for home and office calls is limited to $75 in any one year and the total allowance to an individual member to $350 per year. Family dependents are allowed full payment of charges for office calls and $3.00 toward home calls, laboratory fees, and

X-ray examinations except for dental examinations, with a maximum of $75 per family in any one calendar year.

The persons eligible for benefits are free to select their own physicians and dentists. The association makes direct payment to those who have rendered service to plan members, paying the prevailing fees. The dues and assessments cover disability as well as medical and hospital benefits and are deducted from the weekly wages. The weekly rates for employees are $0.40, $0.45, $0.55, and $0.65, depending upon the earnings, and those for coverage of family dependents are $0.50. The company matches the contributions of the employees on a dollar-for-dollar basis.

Administrative responsibility is vested in a board of trustees appointed by the president of the company and a board of governors elected by the plan members. An "association physician" assists the board in their investigation of claims. The company bears the entire cost of administration.

NONPROFIT PLANS SPONSORED BY MEDICAL SOCIETIES

The cash indemnity plans sponsored by local and state medical societies are established and operated as nonprofit organizations and administered by special agencies created for this purpose. All but a few make payments directly to the physicians.

History and trends of development.—Nearly all the organizations in operation in 1947 were incorporated in the forties. Among the exceptions are the United Medical Service in New York City; Medical and Surgical Care, Inc., in Utica, New York; and the Western New York Medical Plan, Inc., in Buffalo, New York. The United Medical Service was organized in New York in 1944 as successor to a similar plan dating back to 1941 and had 405,726 participants at the end of 1946. Medical and Surgical Care in Utica was organized in 1939 and had an enrollment of 69,429 persons at the end of 1946. The Western New York Medical Plan in Buffalo was established in 1940 and reported 100,281 participants at the end of 1946. The

84 Cash Indemnity Plans

last two originally offered service contracts but later, because of disappointing experiences, dropped them in favor of cash indemnity benefits.

In the early forties several Blue Cross plans began to offer cash indemnity for surgical expenses through riders attached to the hospital service contracts. This step was taken by the Hospital Saving Association of North Carolina and the Intercoast Hospitalization Insurance Association in Sacramento, California, in 1941; the Group Hospital Service of Delaware, the Hospital Care Association of North Carolina, and the Hospital Service of California in 1943; the Hospital Service Association of New Orleans, Louisiana, and the Hospital Service Corporation of Alabama in 1945; and others.

Simultaneously local medical societies began to assume responsibility for the establishment of independent plans. Among them were the Medical Service Association, Durham, North Carolina (1940), the Medical Service, Charleston, West Virginia (1942), and the Community Surgical and Medical Care Plan, Toledo, Ohio (1944). The latter had the benefits underwritten by commercial insurance carriers.

Examples of pioneering state medical societies are those of Pennsylvania, Nebraska, and New Hampshire and Vermont. The first backed the Medical Service Association of Pennsylvania, which was organized in 1940 as a nonprofit corporation providing for cash indemnity benefits as well as service. The latter three were instrumental in establishing straight cash indemnity plans in 1944. The Nebraska Medical Service was organized in the form of a nonprofit assessment insurance company and the New Hampshire–Vermont Physicians' Service as a nonprofit corporation. In 1945, the Ohio State Medical Association sponsored Ohio Medical Indemnity, Inc., organized as a stock insurance company under the insurance laws of the state, and the Missouri State Medical Association organized the Missouri Medical Service under the general nonprofit corporation laws of the state. In 1946, the State Medical Society of Wisconsin put into operation the "Wisconsin Plan," which utilized casualty insurance companies for underwriting purposes.

Finally a number of medical societies endorsed plans offering both cash indemnity benefits for persons earning more than a stated amount and service contracts for participants with incomes below the limit.

As the disparity in the form of organization indicates, no definite pattern has emerged yet. The only fairly discernible trend up to 1947 was that toward state-wide rather than local organization. Accurate figures on the number and enrollment of straight cash indemnity plans are missing. At the end of 1946, thirty-one such organizations were listed by the Council on Medical Service of the American Medical Association [6] and from 60 to 100 per cent of all eligible physicians in the areas covered were participating.

Legal aspects.—Establishment and operation of nonprofit plans providing for cash indemnity is subject to compliance with special state statutes or the state laws governing insurance.

Enabling legislation recently adopted in some states is characterized by two important features, the restriction imposed on incorporation and the permission to combine reimbursement for physicians' bills with hospital service agreements. The Ohio law of 1941, which authorizes nonprofit corporations to operate nonprofit prepayment plans for medical care, requires participation of at least 51 per cent of the duly licensed physicians and surgeons residing and actively practicing in each county where the plan operates,[7] and the New Hampshire law of 1945 stipulates that at least 50 per cent of the eligible physicians in the state or the area of operation must sign up.[8] Several states, such as Alabama, California, Delaware, Louisiana, and North Carolina, have enacted laws permitting hospital service plans to combine provisions for physicians' services with hospitalization contracts. New York amended its statutes in 1946 to provide that "a hospital service corporation and a medical expense indemnity corporation and a dental expense indemnity corporation or any two of such corporations may issue a combined contract providing for hospital care, medical expense indemnity or dental expense indemnity" with the qualification that "no one of such corporations shall issue any such combined contract." [9]

Eligibility requirements.—In general the plans accept employed persons and their family dependents, including the wife (or the husband) and unmarried children between three months and eighteen years of age, provided they enroll in groups of a certain size. Usually a certain proportion of all persons in a potential group of subscribers is required to join.

The minimum percentages vary widely, as the following examples illustrate. One plan requires 60 per cent of a unit of fifty employees or more to sign up, another one at least 30 per cent of the County Farm Bureau membership, and a third one groups of at least five persons from the same place of employment.

In a number of instances eligibility is restricted to persons enrolled in Blue Cross plans. Preliminary physical examination is not a prerequisite, but frequently the applicants must sign a statement that none of the persons whose names appear on the application form has any condition requiring medical or surgical treatment or is under the care of a physician. Age limits are uncommon if the applicants belong to such organizations as nonprofit hospital service plans or farm organizations but are often applied in other cases. Income limits are rarely observed for enrollment but often used to draw a demarcation line between subscribers entitled to reimbursement without additional payments and subscribers who may be charged by the attending physicians for any difference between the allowance and the doctor's usual fee. The United Medical Service in New York City, for instance, in 1947 confined the right to full payment, as stated in the contract, to single persons with a total annual income of less than $1,800 and to married persons with a total annual family income not exceeding $2,500. The Medical Service Association of Pennsylvania relates the income limit to the number of dependent persons in the family. The ceiling in 1947 was $3,120 per year for subscribers with two or more dependents. Persons who leave the original group may retain their membership under certain conditions or transfer to another organization.

Individual enrollment is permitted by a few plans. Persons enrolled through "special application" must be under a certain age, usually under sixty-five years, and pay directly to the plan at rates higher than those charged for "payroll deduction groups."

Reimbursement for the cost of certain types of treatment is subject to waiting periods. These range from nine to twelve months for maternity service, from three to twelve months for removal of tonsils and adenoids, and up to twelve months for hemorrhoid operation, hernia operation, treatment of "menopausal conditions," and treatment of "known pre-existing diseases or ailments." The Missouri Medical Service, for instance, excludes during the first membership year treatment for "arthritis, cancer, diabetes, chronic nephritis, poliomyelitis, osteomyelitis, coronary ailments, congenital deformities, or tuberculosis where condition existed prior to or at the time of application for membership."

Type of illness covered.—Indemnity is usually paid for treatment of diseases and accidents not covered by Workmen's Compensation acts or other local, state, or federal laws and often also for conditions resulting from pregnancy or delivery. It is not allowed for plastic operations for cosmetic purposes and a varying number of other conditions specified in the contracts. Many plans, such as Medical and Surgical Care, Utica, do not honor bills for treatment of "any condition, disease or ailment existing prior to the effective date of the contract."

Type and scope of benefits.—According to the type of benefits, the profession-sponsored cash indemnity plans may be classified in two broad categories: those providing for surgical benefits only and those including medical (nonsurgical) as well as surgical benefits in their scope.

Of the organizations limiting indemnity to surgical expenses, all but a few pay for general surgical services in the hospital and outside. Pertinent examples are the Group Hospital Service of Delaware and the Louisiana Physicians' Service.

Reimbursement for the cost of nonsurgical treatment is limited to care rendered in the hospital in some instances, as in the case of the Hospital Service of California and the Medical Service Association of Pennsylvania. It is extended to include treatment at the home, office, and hospital in other instances, such as Medical and Surgical Care, Utica, New York, and the New Hampshire–Vermont Physicians' Service.

Occasionally several contracts with different benefits are offered. This policy is followed by the United Medical Service in New York City and a few other plans.

Certain auxiliary services, primarily diagnostic X-ray examinations and anesthesia, are covered often and additional ones not infrequently. However, they are always subject to a limit of indemnification per year. The Missouri Medical Service, for instance, allows up to $25 per contract year for diagnostic X-ray procedures, from $5 to $10 for anesthesia, and up to $10 per contract year each for physiotherapy, clinical pathology, surgical pathology, basal metabolism, and electrocardiogram.

Indemnification is made according to a special schedule, printed in a folder or in the subscriber's certificate, or on the basis of a decision by the administration if the services are not listed in the schedule. There is always a maximum indemnity set for specified services and for the total amount reimbursable during a certain period. Family dependents receive the same benefits as breadwinners.

The benefits allowed by the Missouri Medical Service range

from $3.00 for a hospital visit to $150.00 for certain operations such as removal of a kidney, thyroidectomy, or abdominoperineal rectum resection. The surgical benefits are limited to $150 a member year for any one condition and the total value of service per member year to a maximum of $400 for an individual, $900 for two persons, and $1,400 for a family. Medical and Surgical Care, Utica, limits the total benefits allowed under the surgical and medical contracts in each contract year to $225 for any gainfully employed person, $125 for one enrolled dependent, and $350 for three or more enrolled persons in any one family.

In general, bills for treatment of nonsurgical conditions are paid at the rate of $2.00 to $3.00 for hospital visits up to a specified number, at the rate of $2.00 to $2.50 for office visits, and at the rate of $3.00 to $4.00 for home calls.

In 1946, the Hospital Service Corporation of Alabama paid $2.00 for each hospital visit up to a total of 25 visits per year. Medical and Surgical Care, Utica, New York, allowed $2.00 per visit up to a total of 21 for each hospital stay, $2.00 for an office call, and $3.00 each for three home calls within ten days after hospital discharge. The maximum number of reimbursable calls in any one contract year was 48 for a subscriber or dependent and 150 for subscriber and family dependents together. The New Hampshire–Vermont Physicians' Service paid $2.50 for office visits and $3.00 for ordinary home or hospital visits after the second visit. The limit was set at 30 visits per participant in any one year. The Medical Service Association of Pennsylvania reimbursed for costs of nonsurgical treatment in the hospital at the rate of $5.00 per day for the first two days and $3.00 per day for each additional day up to a total of 21 days during the first subscription year, 24 days during the second, 27 days during the third, and 30 days during the fourth and succeeding subscription years. The United Medical Service in New York City under the "surgical-medical plan" allowed $3.00 per day from the fourth day of hospitalization through the twenty-first day and $10.00 per week thereafter up to a total of 111 days. Under the more expensive "general medical plan," additional benefits were paid as follows: $2.00 for office visits and $3.00 for home visits up to a total of twenty visits for any single injury, illness, or pregnancy. In 1947, the allowances were slightly raised by some plans, such as Medical and Surgical Care, Utica.

Organization of professional services.—In contrast to the commercial plans, the medical-society sponsored organizations make definite agreements with doctors of medicine to render service to the subscribers and their dependents. The right to apply for participation is usually extended to all duly licensed physicians practicing in the area of the plan. Physicians who have entered into an agreement with the plan consent to observe the terms of the contract, including the fee schedule, in treating members of the organization. For services covered by the plan they receive payment directly from the administrative office, on proof of services rendered and at the rates set forth in the fee schedule. Only a few plans, such as Ohio Medical Indemnity, make remittances to the subscribers. In many instances the participating physicians are authorized to require additional payments from subscribers with incomes beyond a stipulated limit.

Nonparticipating physicians are paid either the full allowance or a certain proportion only. They are not bound by the rules governing the fees.

Prepayment rates.—The prepayment rates are usually scaled according to the scope of the service offered, the size of the family, and the type of enrollment. In some instances they are also related to the amount of benefits available during a year. As a general rule, they are lower for participants paying through payroll deduction and higher for those who pay directly to the plan.

The United Medical Service in New York City early in

Cash Indemnity Plans

1947 charged monthly rates ranging from $0.40 for one person to $1.80 for a family enrolled in the surgical plan; from $0.64 to $2.36 for one person and a family, respectively, enrolled in the surgical-medical plan; and from $1.60 to $4.00 for coverage by the general medical plan. These rates applied to payroll deduction groups. Participants enrolled through special application were charged quarterly rates ranging from $1.50 to $6.25 for the surgical plan and from $2.50 to $8.50 for the surgical-medical plan.

Medical and Surgical Care, Utica, New York, in 1946 charged group subscribers monthly rates ranging from $0.75 for one person to $1.90 for a typical family enrolled in the surgical plan and from $0.40 to $1.00 for one person and a typical family, respectively, subscribing for medical expense benefits. Under individual enrollment, quarterly rates ranging from $2.25 to $5.70 were charged for surgical benefits and from $1.20 to $3.00 for medical expense benefits. In 1947, slight reductions were made in the cost of the medical expense contract.

The Missouri Medical Service early in 1947 charged monthly rates of $0.85 for individual employees, $1.85 for an employee and one dependent, and $2.25 for family membership, the only plan including maternity benefits. Participants belonging to and paying through County Farm Bureaus were charged quarterly rates ranging from $2.25 for an individual to $6.75 for a family.

Administration.—Administrative responsibility is vested in special agencies. Usually a board of trustees (or directors), serving without remuneration, is given power to lay down the general policies, supervise the operation of the plan, and decide on reimbursement for services not listed in the schedule. Physicians constitute the majority of the trustees or, in some instances, are the only board members. In addition to the board there are appointed officers. The Missouri Medical Service, for instance, has a board of sixteen trustees—including twelve physicians and four representatives of the general public—and five officers, of whom three are members of the medical profession.

As a rule, paid executive and clerical personnel is employed for the management of the plans. Their number depends largely on the degree of cooperation with Blue Cross plans, which in a number of instances carry out certain tasks, especially enrollment and specified business procedures.

Approval.—Approval by the Council on Medical Service and Public Relations of the American Medical Association is given to those plans which meet the standards of acceptance set forth by the Council. As the benefits of acceptable plans "may be in terms of cash indemnity," [19] many profession-sponsored plans of this type have obtained approval and with it the right to display the "seal of acceptance."

The utilization of commercial insurance companies by some profession-sponsored plans has posed a serious problem. Should commercial carriers be admitted to participation in medical society plans? If the answer is affirmative, what conditions should be set for cooperation and, with it, for approval?

FIVE

Nonprofit Hospital Service Plans: Blue Cross Plans

ALL nonprofit hospital service plans are alike in their general objectives and basic policies. They are designed to make hospitalization more easily available by substituting group payment for individual obligations. They establish and administer common funds into which subscribers make regular prepayments and from which the costs of hospitalization are paid in full or in part. The subscribers, the hospitals, and the administrative agencies accept certain duties and have clearly defined rights.

The large majority of the nonprofit hospital service plans in operation at present are "free-choice plans" providing service through most of the hospitals in a local community or a state. Organizations sponsored by single hospitals in a community, important as they originally were in their areas, now play a relatively minor role in number, membership, and volume of service rendered and therefore will be omitted from the following presentation.

Basic principles.—Blue Cross plans are community-sponsored nonprofit corporations organized to furnish specified types and amounts of hospital services to persons making regular and equal prepayments. Their operation is based on contracts with both subscribers and hospitals. Their form of organization places them in the position of an intermediary agency representing the interests of both the hospitals and the public.[1]

The distinctive feature of Blue Cross plans is the guarantee of service. "The benefits of a non-profit hospital service plan are assured by the member hospitals through definite contractual agreements which are equitable and consistent with respect to the rights and obligations of the subscribers, the plan, and the hospitals." [2] The members of a plan usually have free choice of "member hospitals." In some instances they may select any hospital. The hospitals receive agreed rates of payment from the agency administering the plan.

The principle of offering service rather than cash indemnity was adopted by the Blue Cross plans from the outset. As the standards issued by the American Hospital Association in 1938 stated: "Benefits to subscribers should be guaranteed through 'service' contracts with member hospitals as opposed to 'cash' indemnification contracts for hospital expense." [3] This principle was defined in more detail in the Association's revised standards of 1942 as follows: "Benefits in member hospitals should be expressed in 'service contracts,' which describe specifically the types and amounts of hospital services to which the subscribers are entitled." [4] Reaffirming its old policy, the Blue Cross Commission of the American Hospital Association in March, 1946, passed a resolution that "Blue Cross Plans in which member hospitals do not provide benefits on a service basis be asked to show cause why approval should be continued by the American Hospital Association." The approval program as revised in September, 1946, states: "Member hospitals are urged to cooperate with Blue Cross Plans in providing complete hospital care as service benefits under the subscribers' contracts." [5]

History and trends of development.—In 1929, a group of school teachers in Dallas, Texas, made a contract with the Baylor University Hospital. Each teacher agreed to pay $3.00 per semester, and the hospital in turn consented to furnish up to three weeks of hospitalization in semiprivate accommodations with no extra charges for the use of the operating room, for laboratory services, and for routine drugs and dressings. This plan is credited with having been the spark that kindled Blue Cross plans, although similar plans had been established before in various communities such as Rockford, Illinois (1912), Grinnell, Iowa (1921), and Brattleboro, Vermont (1927).

Significantly, it was the economic depression of the thirties that stimulated the development of nonprofit hospital service plans. In 1933, the American Hospital Association went on record in favor of such plans, and in 1934 the American College of Surgeons passed a pertinent resolution at its annual meeting, after its Board of Regents had approved a detailed report by the Medical Service Board on "principles which should be observed in the development and conduct of prepayment plans for medical and hospital service."[6] Between 1933 and 1937, a small number of plans were established. By the end of 1937, there were thirty-nine plans in operation and their membership had risen beyond one million. In 1946 the national enrollment passed the twenty million mark. Substantial further growth since is indicated by the latest figures. Details are given on page 97. One of the major factors contributing to this remarkable development was the high income of many socioeconomic groups in the early forties. Up to 1941, "breadwinners" accounted for the majority of all participants, but since the early forties family dependents have constituted the largest group, numerically and proportionately. The number of individuals per contract increased from 1.80 in 1939 to 2.25 in 1945 and 2.27 on January 1, 1947. Significantly about six tenths of the total membership on January 1, 1947 was enrolled in fourteen plans with more than 500,000 members each.

Many of the early plans originally were designed to serve local communities but later expanded to cover the entire area of their states. Most of the more recent plans started out as state-wide organizations. As of January 1, 1947, there were twenty-seven Blue Cross plans operating on a state-wide basis, and one plan each in the District of Columbia and in Puerto Rico.

The geographic expansion was stimulated and facilitated by the tendency to include Blue Cross service in collective bargaining agreements between management and labor unions; to enroll farmers through units of the American Farm Bureau Federation, the National Grange, the Farmers Union, and other organizations; and to utilize Blue Cross plans for the purpose of furnishing hospitalization to persons covered by general prepayment plans for medical care, such as cooperative health service associations, or to members of employee mutual benefit associations.

On January 1, 1947, about 19 per cent of the total population of the United States was enrolled in Blue Cross plans. In some states a substantial fraction of the population had been reached: 66.3 per cent in Rhode Island, 48.7 per cent in Massachusetts, and 47.2 per cent in Delaware. The Cleveland Hospital Service Association had enrolled close to 70 per cent of all the people living in the counties covered.

The development in New York State is interesting from various points of view. In that state, hospitalization insurance

ENROLLMENT IN APPROVED HOSPITAL SERVICE PLANS IN THE UNITED STATES *

	NUMBER OF PLANS	ENROLLMENT
Jan. 1, 1938	39	1,364,975
Jan. 1, 1939	53	2,874,055
Jan. 1, 1940	55	4,409,593
Jan. 1, 1941	65	6,012,483
Jan. 1, 1942	66	8,399,433
Jan. 1, 1943	74	10,215,241
Jan. 1, 1944	73	12,600,205
Jan. 1, 1945	76	15,771,594
Jan. 1, 1946	81	18,898,779
Jan. 1, 1947	82	24,283,173

* Figures supplied by the Blue Cross Commission of the American Hospital Association. The approval system went into effect in 1938.

Blue Cross Plans

was first tried out in New York City in 1935. Within the next few years eight other plans were organized. At the end of 1935 there were 64,139 persons enrolled, 40,439 in the New York City plan and 23,700 in the Rochester plan. By July, 1945, the nine plans had 3,158,145 participants, thus serving 22.7 per cent of the population of the state; the plan in Rochester had boosted its enrollment to a figure equal to 47.6 per cent of the population of its area.[7]

With the growth of Blue Cross plans, the number of participating hospitals has increased markedly. On October 1, 1944, a total of 2,959 hospitals with 308,365 beds were on the roster of member hospitals in the United States, and of these 8.9 per cent were governmental, 17.3 per cent proprietary, 64.7 per cent nonprofit voluntary, and 9.1 per cent unclassified. Of the total bed capacity in all member hospitals, 78.7 per cent was in nonprofit voluntary hospitals, 11.4 per cent in governmental hospitals, 6.4 per cent in proprietary hospitals, and 3.5 per cent in unclassified facilities.[8]

ROLE OF THE AMERICAN HOSPITAL ASSOCIATION

Since 1933 the American Hospital Association has been playing an important role in the development of Blue Cross plans. It has promoted the movement, guided it into proper channels, formulated standards for nonprofit hospital service plans, introduced the approval system, and emphasized the establishment of satisfactory working relations between hospitals and Blue Cross administrations and between medical service and hospital service plans.

As early as 1933, a booklet "Essentials of an Acceptable Plan of Group Hospitalization" was issued. In 1937, a special committee, later known as the Hospital Service Plan Commission, was established and authorized to recommend formal approval of nonprofit hospital service plans. The approval program was initiated in 1938 on the basis of "Standards for Non-Profit Hospital Care Insurance Plans" and became the direct responsibility of the Board of Trustees of the American Hospital Association in 1941. As Article VIII, Section 6 of the bylaws of this organization states:

The Board of Trustees shall establish standards for and administer a program of annual approval for organizations operating nonprofit hospital service plans which apply for such approval. The purpose of the standards shall be to protect the interests of the subscribers, the medical profession, and the hospitals.

Leaning on the experience gained in the past, the Board of Trustees on June 29, 1946, approved a set of principles defining the relationship of hospitals and Blue Cross plans.[9]

Since 1946, the responsibility for the various tasks involved, in particular for the coordination of all plans, administrative counsel, consumer education, and collection and distribution of statistical data, rests with the "Blue Cross Commission," the successor of the "Hospital Service Plan Commission" which in 1941 had been established within the Association to continue the work of earlier committees and subdivisions.

Legal aspects.—Blue Cross plans function under special statutes or the corporation laws of the states. They are differentiated from stock or mutual assessment insurance companies and classed as organizations not subject to the regular insurance laws of the states and their requirements. They are exempted from taxation by the states and localities, being treated like "charitable and benevolent institutions," and from federal income taxes under Section 101 (8) as "organizations for social welfare" but not from responsibility for meeting the requirements of the Social Security Act of 1935. Usually they are regulated and supervised by the insurance departments of the states.

Following the lead of New York State, which passed the first "enabling act" in 1934, the majority of the states adopted special legislation governing the organization and supervision of nonprofit hospital service plans. By July, 1946, such laws had been passed by thirty-six states. A small number of states have ruled, through their attorneys general or departments of insurance, that nonprofit hospital service plans are permitted to operate under the general corporation laws.

The enabling act passed in Michigan in 1939 contains the following clause:

Any number of persons, not less than 7, may form a corporation, under and in conformity with the provisions of this act, for the purpose of establishing, maintaining and operating a non-profit hospital service plan, whereby hospital service may be provided by any hospital or group of hospitals with which such corporation has a contract for such purpose, to such of the public as become subscribers to said plan under a contract with such corporation which entitles each subscriber to certain hospital care. Any such non-profit hospital service corporation shall be subject to regulation and supervision by the commissioner of insurance . . .[10]

The enabling acts vary considerably in detail but have certain elements in common.[11] In many states they prohibit hospital service from providing any medical or surgical services in violation of the acts governing the practice of medicine.

In an effort to bring about more uniformity of legislation, the American Hospital Association has proposed a model law.[12] Despite the efforts of this association and despite the passage of acts by most states, the legal basis of Blue Cross plans is still in the formative stage. Amendments to the state statutes were made often in recent years, and more may be adopted in the near future.

Eligibility requirements.—Group enrollment of employed persons is either required or strongly emphasized, and eligibility is usually extended to the dependent spouse and to children up to nineteen years of age. At the end of 1946, this limit was in force in fifty-six plans. The minimum age at which newborn children are eligible varies widely, ranging from the time of birth in many instances to three months in many others and more than three months in a few cases only. In the early stage, only large groups were permitted to join, but lately groups consisting of as few as five or fewer persons at one place of employment have been accepted by the majority of the plans.

Individual enrollment, recommended by a special committee of the Blue Cross Commission in 1944, was permitted by about half the plans at the end of 1946. It is promoted by various devices, in particular "community enrollment" campaigns conducted for a limited period of time, usually a month. Carrying this principle farther, about forty plans in twenty-three states participated in a coordinated program of enrollment of veterans and their families during a one-month period in 1946. In general, "non-group subscribers" have obligations and rights differing from those of group subscribers. In some instances they pay higher rates for the regular services or for more restricted benefits; in others they pay the usual, somewhat higher, "direct pay rates" and are eligible for all or many of the regular services.

Persons qualifying for enrollment according to the general policy of the plans are accepted without preliminary medical examinations and regardless of the size of their earnings. They receive needed service without a waiting period, except for maternity care, which usually is provided after nine or more months of continuous membership.

Age limits for new members enrolling in groups are applied by the minority of all plans. Nearly all of some thirty plans which at the end of 1946 did use a limit had set it at sixty-five years of age. In contrast, original enrollment of "non-group" applicants is limited by the large majority of the plans to persons under sixty-five years of age and by a few to persons under seventy years.

Subscribers and their eligible dependents who leave the place of employment through which they have been enrolled may transfer to another plan or continue their membership through "direct payment," usually in quarterly amounts.

Types of illness covered.—As a general rule, Blue Cross service is available for all but a small number of specified types of disease and injury and for maternity care. It always excludes accidents and diseases covered by Workmen's Compensation acts or other laws. Other exclusions vary widely. In 1946 about one third of all plans did not cover service for conditions which existed on the effective date of the membership certificate or for which medical attention had been received within a stipulated period prior to such date. In addition, treatment of certain diseases, such as communicable diseases, mental deviations, and drug and alcohol addiction, was barred completely or limited to a specified number of days by a considerable number of plans, and admission solely for diagnosis was excluded by more than half.

Type and scope of service.—The basic services to which plan members are entitled include board and room, general nursing care, use of the operating and delivery room, specified laboratory services, and routine medications and dressings. Full service is furnished for at least twenty-one to thirty days in any one contract year. Many plans make provisions for semiprivate service only, others for ward as well as semiprivate service, and some for ward service only. The prepayment rates are adjusted accordingly. Dependents receive benefits equivalent to those of subscribers in the majority of all instances. Regardless of the type of accommodation, Blue Cross members are expected to pay their attending physicians.

Frequently the hospital benefits go much beyond the scope of the basic services. A considerable number of plans offer also special diets, anesthesia, basal metabolism examinations, emergency room service, X-ray services, and a variety of other services, and they make all their benefits available for each illness or disability. Nearly all plans allow an additional period during which the subscriber receives half benefits. The following are examples of plans with liberal provisions.

The Michigan Hospital Service, a state-wide plan, at the end of 1946 provided for thirty days of hospitalization and ninety additional days at 50 per cent of the hospital's regular charges. The services included general nursing care; meals and special diets; use of the operating and delivery room; anesthesia by salaried hospital employee, nurse, or lay anesthetist; all laboratory services except electrocardiograms; drugs and dressings; oxygen; physical therapy; basal metabolism examinations; and emergency (accident) room service. These services were available for each disability. Maternity care was subject to a waiting period of nine months which, however, did not apply to abnormal conditions.

The Hospital Service Corporation of Rhode Island, a state-wide plan, at the end of 1946 offered 150 days of hospitalization each contract year, with 75 days for any one cause, under comprehensive enrollment; 62 days each contract year, with 31 days for any one cause, under "standard group" enrollment, that is, enrollment of groups representing less than 90 per cent of the total possible; and 31 days each contract year under the direct payment plan.

The Colorado Hospital Service, a state-wide plan, offered full service for 30 days and 50 per cent discount for 90 additional days. Patients with mental disease and those with tuberculosis were eligible for 30 days of service.

A considerable number of approved hospital service plans is coordinated with prepayment plans for physicians' services. As of January 1, 1947, the number of affiliated medical-surgical plans was 42 and their total enrollment 4,185,827. Participants in Blue Cross plans constitute a large fraction of the membership of medical-society plans. In Utica, for instance, more than half of all the Hospital Plan members also subscribe to the "Surgical and Special Benefit Plan" of Medical and Surgical Care, Inc.

All plans allow for benefits in cases of emergencies arising in communities without member hospitals. As a general rule, the subscriber receives a fixed sum per day as allowance toward his expenditures, the amount differing for ward and semiprivate service, for subscribers and family dependents, and for short and long stay.

Many Blue Cross plans cooperate with one another by readily accepting subscribers who move from the community where they have been enrolled to another one served by a plan and by furnishing service to members falling sick while away from their residence. Early in 1947, more than forty plans in the United States were participating in an "Inter-Plan Service Benefit Agreement."

Prepayment rates.—The prepayment rates, also called "subscription fees" or "premiums," differ slightly from plan to plan. They vary according to the type of service (ward or semiprivate), the size of the family, the method of enrollment (individual or group enrollment), and the method of collection (payroll deduction or direct payment from the subscriber to the plan).

In 1946, the monthly prepayment rates under group enrollment ranged from $0.50 to $1.25 for single persons and from $1.00 to $3.60 for families subscribing to ward service; and from $0.65 to $1.40 for single persons and from $1.30 to $3.30 for families subscribing to semiprivate service. The rates for persons joining under the system of individual enrollment were somewhat higher. In 1947, all rates were increased by many plans.

The Michigan Hospital Service at the end of 1946 charged group subscribers to the ward service plan monthly prepayment rates of $1.12 for single persons and $2.60 for families, including all dependent children. The rates for the semiprivate service plan were $1.40 for single persons and $3.10 for families, including all dependent children.

The Associated Hospital Service of New York City, the

largest in the country, early in 1947 charged the following rates: $0.80 monthly for a single person, $1.60 for a couple, and $2.00 for a family enrolled under group contract; $2.60, $5.20, and $6.60 quarterly or $10.00, $20.00, and $26.00 annually for individual subscribers, couples, and families, respectively, who paid directly or were accepted on the basis of "special applications." All rates apply to semiprivate service.

In recent years a growing number of private employers and public agencies have contributed to the cost of Blue Cross services by paying part or all of the subscription fees for their employees and in some instances also for the family dependents. The Associated Hospital Service of New York, for instance, at the end of 1946 listed a total of 3,617 firms which were paying on behalf of nearly 470,000 plan members, with a substantial proportion of the companies contributing for family dependents as well as employees. The same policy has been adopted by a number of city governments, such as Chattanooga, Tennessee; Detroit, Michigan; and Sapulpa, Oklahoma; and by the Insular Government of Puerto Rico.

Methods of paying hospitals.—In paying hospitals for services rendered to Blue Cross subscribers, the plans follow different methods. Some pay a flat rate to all hospitals or groups of them. Others pay rates with some relation to cost and with modifications in different areas. Still others pay at established rates for accommodations occupied, with variations according to locality.[13]

Administrative organization.—The typical Blue Cross plan is administered by a policy-making and supervising board of directors (or trustees) whose members serve without remuneration and a paid staff of executive and other personnel. The board is composed of representatives of the participating hospitals, the medical profession, and the general public. The proportionate distribution of seats varies greatly. In many instances, representatives of the hospitals and the medical profession constitute the majority. As the standards of the American Hospital Association declare, "The interests and the responsibilities of participating hospitals make it desirable that a majority of the policy-making body be hospital trustees, administrators, and/or authorized representatives of the member hospitals." [14]

The paid staff usually includes an executive director and a varying number of other executive, supervisory, and clerical personnel. The major administrative units are the enrollment, contract, hospital record, comptroller's, actuarial and statistical, purchasing and supply, publicity, tabulating, mailing, and personnel departments.

The Hospital Service Corporation of Rhode Island at the end of 1946 had a total of 79 full-time employees to handle the accounts of 466,000 participants, or one employee for every 5,900 participants.[15]

In addition to a board of directors, some plans, such as the Cleveland Hospital Service Association, have an advisory committee of hospital administrators who advise on matters pertaining to the administration of hospitals and may initiate recommendations to the board.

Realizing that public acceptance and subscriber participation in the formulation of policies are vital to successful operation, Blue Cross plans have lately taken steps to organize subscriber councils selected from the leaders of enrolled groups.[16] Among plans adopting this policy were the Hospital Care Corporation, Cincinnati, Ohio; the Kansas Hospital Service Association; the Group Hospital Service, St. Louis, Missouri; and the Blue Cross Hospital Service of Indiana. In Cincinnati, the council is subdivided into "area subscribers' committees."

Many Blue Cross plans are recognized by the Veterans Administration as administrative units for the provision of medical care for veterans with service-connected disabilities. A substantial number have made various arrangements for administrative cooperation with medical service plans organized under the auspices of medical societies.[17]

Approval.—Approval, including permission to use the term "Blue Cross Plan," is given by the Board of Trustees of the American Hospital Association to those nonprofit hospital service plans which meet the standards of the Association. The requirements for original approval specify details as to adequate representation of the hospitals, the medical profession, and the general public in the administration; nonprofit sponsorship and control; free choice of hospital and physician; hospital responsibility for benefits to subscribers; enrollment areas and practices; sound accounting practices; adequate reserves; adequate statistical records; equitable payments to hospitals; dignified promotion and administration; and inter-plan coordination. Reapproval is subject to compliance with standards set for this purpose.[18]

Experience.—The vast experience gained since the late thirties has greatly improved the knowledge of the technical factors that make or break nonprofit hospital service plans. Moreover, it has yielded useful information on the value of the basic policies and procedures followed. The Blue Cross Commission of the American Hospital Association has regularly published actuarial tables prepared from data submitted by approved plans.[19]

The major lessons learned in regard to underwriting and administration have been summarized as follows. Women use more service than men, older people require more care than younger persons, subscribers who have left their place of employment need more care than before, and various occupational groups differ in their demand for service. Obstetrical care is a significant part of the cost of any health insurance plan. The size of the prepayment rates determines both the degree of participation within a community and the utilization of benefits. The scope of the program affects the extent to which service is actually used.[20]

Blue Cross Plans

Up to 1941, the subscribers to Blue Cross plans came primarily from the middle and higher income groups and to a relatively small extent from the low income groups. This changed with the increase in the number of plans offering ward service contracts. Where choice between ward and semiprivate service is offered, ward service contracts are taken by a substantial number of subscribers only if the price is appreciably lower and the benefits and privileges are about the same. Ward service contracts implying a means test are unpopular. In 1944, the percentage of participants with ward service contracts was 46.4 in the Hospital Service Association of Toledo, 45.1 in the Michigan Hospital Service, 19.5 in the Hospital Service Corporation of Rhode Island, and 17.4 in the Hospital Service Association of Northeastern Pennsylvania.

The number of people in rural areas who are reached by Blue Cross plans is insignificant. By the middle of 1946, only 2.65 per cent of the rural population was enrolled as contrasted to 27 per cent of the urban population.

The median number of hospital admissions per 1,000 participants in various groups of reporting plans was 107 in 1941, 108 in 1942, 106 in 1943, 103 in 1944, 107 in 1945, and 111 in 1946. The rate was relatively highest in plans with less than 50,000 participants and relatively lowest in plans with 500,000 or more members.

The median number of patient days per eligible person was 0.81 in 1941, 0.83 in 1942, 0.79 in 1943, 0.80 in 1944, 0.84 in 1945, and 0.84 in 1946. The median length of stay of the hospitalized patient was 7.60 days in 1941, 7.80 days in 1942, 7.83 days in 1943, 7.78 days in 1944, 7.56 days in 1945, and 8.30 days in 1946.

The major causes of hospitalized illness, as reported by seventeen plans, were diseases of the respiratory system and diseases of the digestive system, which together accounted for nearly four tenths of all admissions. Deliveries ranked next in frequency. These three groups accounted for 56.4 per cent of all admissions and approximately one half of all hospital days, deliveries requiring nearly one fifth of all days.[21]

The median cost per hospitalized case as reported by various groups of plans amounted to $48.55 in 1944, $47.69 in 1945, and $52.63 in 1946. In Michigan the average payments made by the Blue Cross plan were $61.00 per patient in 1944, $58.53 in 1945, and $64.61 in 1946. In Cleveland, they were $61.85 in 1945 and $66.01 in 1946.

The average expense for hospital care per patient day (median for all groups of plans) was $5.59 in 1940, $6.00 in 1944, and $5.21 in 1945. It must be borne in mind that some plans provide only ward service and others semi-private as well as ward service. In Michigan the average payment per patient day was $7.39 in 1944, $7.16 in 1945, and $7.81 in 1946.

A sample study of five Blue Cross plans in the state of New York showed that in 1944 most bills for semiprivate service were under $100 and that Blue Cross plans paid from 50 per cent to 90 per cent of the hospital charges to plan members in cases covered by the contract, the proportion being relatively highest when the total bill was low.[22] In Michigan, in 1944, Blue Cross patients received hospital care in the amount of $7,509,859. Of this sum, $5,818,827 was paid by the plan and $1,691,032 by the patients for services not covered by their contracts.[23]

The total income of Blue Cross plans was $46,300,000 in 1941, $62,200,000 in 1942, $76,900,000 in 1943, $96,900,000 in 1944, $128,700,000 in 1945, and $171,700,000 in 1946. The median income per contract in various groups of reporting plans was $13.21 in 1941, $13.98 in 1942, $13.84 in 1943, $14.39 in 1944, $14.82 in 1945, and $16.47 in 1946. The corresponding figures for income per participant were $6.46, $6.51, $6.14, $6.39, $6.77, and $6.94. Of the 1941 income, 70.52 per cent was used to pay the participating hospitals, 12.29 per cent to cover operating expenses, and 17.19 per cent to build up contingency reserves. In 1945, the picture was different. Of the total income, 81.38 per cent was spent on hospital care and 12.29 per cent on operating expenses, while 6.33 per cent was put in reserve.[24] The administrative costs of the plans varied with the size of membership, tending to be relatively lowest in plans with large enrollment. The Cleveland Hospital Service Association, for instance, reported slightly more than 7 per cent administrative expenses in each of the years 1944, 1945, and 1946.[25]

Payments from Blue Cross plans have come to constitute an important source of income for the participating hospitals. A study conducted in Michigan in 1944 revealed that 22.7 per cent of all patient days recorded by the general hospitals in Wayne County were paid for by the Michigan Hospital Service. In Rhode Island in 1946 the participating hospitals derived from 40 to 50 per cent of their income from Blue Cross payments.[26] Already in 1941, when the national enrollment figure was still small, the amount paid out to nongovernmental hospitals represented about 10 per cent of their total income, thus exceeding "the combined receipts from endowment income and community fund contributions for hospitalization." [27] In 1945, payments from Blue Cross plans were estimated to constitute more than one fourth of the hospital income from patients.

The number of full-time employees of thirty-five Blue Cross plans, representing 37 per cent of the total membership, averaged 0.33 per 1,000 members in April, 1947.[28]

Achievements.—Blue Cross plans have proved to be of considerable value to the patients, the participating hospitals, and the practicing physicians.

A hospital bill "involves a severe physical shock, a high emotional crisis, and a large economic expenditure." [29] The programs serve to remove a source of grave anxiety and to lighten the financial burden of hospitalization. They enable the sick to receive hospital service earlier, more frequently, and in larger amount than would have been possible without organized group prepayment. The patients appreciate both the sense of security and the tangible advantages obtained by membership in a plan. Those who belong to the middle income group, as most of them do, are hospitalized about twice as often as persons of the same income class were in 1929, when the purchasing power of the dollar was considerably higher and prepayment plans were few and far between. What is even more significant, the frequency of hospitalization of Blue Cross members in the early forties has been almost identical with the theoretical standard of adequacy suggested by Roger I. Lee and Lewis W. Jones,[30] which at the end of the twenties were barely reached by families with incomes of $10,000 and more.

Most of the participating hospitals derive noteworthy advantages from their cooperation with Blue Cross plans. As payment for service to plan members is guaranteed, the hospitals receive more patients whose bills are safe, although some are critical of the inadequacy of the rates and a few have withdrawn from Blue Cross plans because of losses. As a prize-winning slogan put it, "Pay patients appreciate hospitals, hospitals appreciate pay patients." The hospital administrations save time and money for bookkeeping and collection of debts and can estimate income and expenses with greater certainty. The remittances from Blue Cross plans constitute a substantial source of income for many hospitals and enable them to maintain and improve their standards of service. Not the least important asset is aptly described in the following phrase: "Blue Cross builds unity between hospitals and community."

The physicians have more freedom in suggesting necessary treatment in a hospital since the economic barrier is reduced; in addition, they can expect the patients to be able to pay for professional services more readily.[31]

From a general point of view, Blue Cross plans are important in several respects. They serve to minimize the risk of illness by facilitating early hospitalization of apparently minor conditions and prompt admission of serious conditions, and they contribute to the reduction of the frequency of dependency caused by high-cost illness. With their growth, public understanding of the prepayment method is improved and interest in its wide application aroused. The policy of limiting the number of plans is conducive to the development of large and financially strong organizations.

Shortcomings.—The Blue Cross service is not perfect, as both friends and critics have stated again and again. Some of the shortcomings of the plans, especially the disparity in the scope, amount, and period of service, may be remedied if determined efforts are made to achieve uniformity of basic contracts. Other defects are inherent in the basic principle of insurance and in the policy followed in its application. They may be alleviated but they cannot be eliminated.

Membership in a Blue Cross plan is accessible only to those who meet the eligibility requirements and feasible only for persons able to pay the rates charged. There are millions of self-supporting individuals and families in all income groups who could not qualify for enrollment, even if liberal requirements were adopted universally. In large and small communities alike, there are tens of millions with low incomes who cannot afford the full prepayments but can make some contributions toward the cost of the service. In rural areas the enrollment poses problems not only because of the inadequacy of net cash incomes but because of the difficulties of reaching people on isolated farms, collecting the prepayments, and guaranteeing service where good hospitals are scarce or far away. Substantial turnover of membership has proved to be one of the serious drawbacks to economical operation of the programs. The widely used slogan "once a member, always a member" presumes not only satisfaction with the service but availability of plans everywhere and ability to pay all the time.

As it stands at present, the Blue Cross program meets only part of the hospital-care needs of the subscribers and their family dependents. Important diseases and defects are entirely or partly excluded from coverage. The total period of full benefits is limited. In a number of instances, the family dependents are entitled only to a fraction of the services available to "breadwinners." Substantial additional expenditures for hospitalization are especially necessary in cases of serious illness. Reciprocity of service is still unsatisfactory because of the variations in both service to patients and rates of payment to hospitals. The goal of "national cohesion" appears far distant. Subscribers hospitalized in "nonmember hospitals" often receive much less than the value of the services available in member hospitals. Admission of inferior hospitals is hard to avoid in areas lacking facilities of high standards.

With a few exceptions, the services of physicians are not covered at all or are made available under separate plans covering selected types of care only. Ample experience has shown that at least one half, if not more, of the average total cost of illness requiring hospitalization goes for professional services in the hospital. There are many who are convinced that merger of hospital and medical service plans into single plans is mandatory lest the professional and economic interdependence of hospital care and professional service be neglected. Moreover, limitation of service to in-patients puts a premium on hospitalization and discourages "extramural" treatment.

The administrative organization of Blue Cross plans has been, and continues to be, the subject of considerable criticism. The lack of adequate subscriber representation is deplored—and resented—on the grounds that "the folks who put up the money" are deprived of the opportunity to participate in the decisions on the use of the premium income. The overhead costs are relatively high, due to the necessity of meeting rather heavy expenses for promotion. The administrative separation of Blue Cross plans from other community health agencies, voluntary as well as governmental, has ac-

Blue Cross Plans

centuated the need for coordination of the activities of the countless organizations administering health services.

Compared with the situation prevailing before the introduction of Blue Cross plans, the service provided by these organizations constitutes a very great improvement. Compared with standards of adequacy, it is deficient. A statement made in 1944 by C. Rufus Rorem, a leader in the development of Blue Cross plans, was still true in 1947: "The Blue Cross plans have exceeded all expectations, but they have not yet realized their full possibilities. Both critics and friends demand a broader and deeper accomplishment, if voluntary group prepayment for hospital service is to serve the needs of the American people." [32]

SIX

Nonprofit Physicians' Service Plans: Blue Shield Plans

THE nonprofit prepayment plans for physicians' service which utilize the system of the individual practice of medicine provide subscribers with specified types of services by those duly licensed and registered physicians who are participating in the program. They operate on the basis of contractual agreements with both subscribers and physicians. The persons covered by the plans are free to choose any of the members of the medical profession whose names are on the roster. The physicians receive direct payment from the administrative agency for such services as are covered by the prepayment plan, at rates fixed by agreement between the two parties.

The service principle is not always maintained. Combination of service and indemnity benefits is offered by some plans and choice between the two types of contracts by others.

Predominant in this category are the Blue Shield plans, nonprofit organizations established and operated under the auspices of medical societies.

History and trends of development.—Nearly all the medical society plans in operation in 1947 were organized after 1938. The majority are state-wide rather than local. This pattern was set by some of the early plans which succeeded in enrolling substantial numbers of participants: the California Physicians' Service (1939), the Michigan Medical Service (1939), and the Massachusetts Medical Service (1942). By the end of 1946, the Michigan Medical Service had 840,961 participants; the Massachusetts Medical Service, 460,514; and the California Physicians' Service, 419,672.

Originally establishment of a separate administrative organization was the rule. Recently cooperation with Blue Cross plans has developed in various forms and to a widely varying degree. The principle of maintaining separate organizations, one for physicians' service and one for hospitalization, has been abandoned in a few instances.

Legal aspects.—Initiation and operation of prepayment plans for physicians' service are regulated by special acts of the states ("enabling acts") or by statutes such as corporation laws.

The challenging objective of enabling legislation is well stated in the laws of Michigan and Massachusetts. The act of the state of Michigan, which was adopted in 1939 to permit and regulate the incorporation of nonprofit medical care corporations, defines its purpose and intent as follows: ". . . to promote a wider distribution of medical care and to maintain the standing and promote the progress of the science and art of medicine . . ." [1] The enabling act of the state of Massachusetts, passed in 1941, "provides for the preservation of the public health by furnishing medical services at low cost to members of the public who become subscribers of the charitable corporations formed [under the act] . . ." [2]

The Michigan law draws a sharp line between a service plan and an organization providing for cash indemnity, by setting forth that "no contract by or on behalf of any non-profit medical care corporation shall provide for the payment of any cash or other material benefit by that corporation to the subscriber or his estate on account of death, illness or injury, nor be in any way related to the payment of any such benefit by any other agency." In addition, it forbids the use of any name including the words "insurance, casualty, surety, health and accident, mutual or other words descriptive of the insurance or surety business."

In a number of states, the laws have been drafted in such a way as to restrict the initiation of nonprofit prepayment plans. The New Jersey law of 1940 states that "no person, firm, association, or corporation other than a medical service corporation shall establish, maintain or operate a medical service plan or any other means, agency or device for contracting with persons to pay for medical services" and, in addition, requires 51 per cent of the eligible physicians in the area of the plan to agree to participate.[3] The Pennsylvania act of 1939 stipulates that the majority of the incorporators must be physicians,[4] and the Minnesota act of 1945 requires "not less than 21 doctors licensed under State laws and legal residents of the State" for purposes of incorporation.[5]

As a general rule, the nonprofit physicians' service plans are not permitted to include hospitalization. They are supervised by the insurance departments of the states, although there are a few exceptions to this rule. In Pennsylvania, for instance, the Medical Service Association is under the joint direction and supervision of the Department of Health and the Department of Insurance. In California, the Supreme Court of that state in 1946 ruled that the California Physicians' Service is not subject to the supervision of the state's Insurance Commissioner.[6]

Eligibility requirements.—In general, the plans require group enrollment, accept only employed persons and their family dependents—defined as wife or husband and unmarried children between the ages of three months and eighteen years—and limit the prepaid services to subscribers earning less than a stated amount a year. In some instances, enrollment is confined to persons holding membership in a Blue Cross plan.

At the end of 1946, groups consisting of as few as five persons from the same place of employment were admitted by some plans, such as those in the states of California, Florida, and Kansas, and in Milwaukee, Wisconsin. Usually a certain percentage of all employees in a given unit had to sign up to make enrollment effective.

Very few plans extend eligibility to self-employed persons, and then only if they are members of organizations cooperating with the plans, apply during the period of a special community-enrollment campaign, or pass a medical examination. The income limits at the end of 1946 ranged from $1,500 for single subscribers and $2,400 for subscribers with families, to $3,000 and $5,000 for single persons and families, respectively. In Massachusetts, beginning on June 1, 1947, the income limits are $2,000 for single subscribers, $2,500 for a couple, and $3,000 for the family with children. Under the North Idaho plan they are $3,000 after taxes for single subscribers and $4,750 for a family of four.

Not infrequently the physicians are authorized to make extra charges for treatment of plan members whose earnings exceed the limit. As the official publication of the American Medical Association explains: "It is recognized that the incomes of persons determine their ability to pay; therefore, for certain income groups the physicians agree to provide the benefits without additional charges. To this extent a contract becomes a service contract." [7] The regular benefits apply, however, regardless of income. In many instances, provisions are made for transfer to other plans or for continuation of membership after a subscriber has left his original group.

Type of illness covered.—The services of the prepayment plans are available for treatment of diseases and injuries and for maternity care not provided by local, state, or federal laws. Mental diseases, tuberculosis, self-inflicted injuries, and plastic operations for cosmetic purposes are usually excluded. There are waiting periods for specified services. They range from nine to twelve months for maternity care, from three to twelve months for elective surgery, such as tonsillectomy and herniotomy, and from nine to twelve months for pre-existing conditions. In recent years a tendency has developed to waive waiting periods for service other than maternity care if at least 75 per cent of a group of eligible persons enroll.

Type and scope of service.—Protection against the "most dramatic expense item" or "catastrophic illness" has been the objective of the plans up to 1947. As a rule, general surgical care, including certain auxiliary services, is provided for hospitalized persons. Physicians' service for inpatients with non-surgical conditions is covered by some programs, and medical service outside the hospital by a few.

The term general surgical care is interpreted as meaning "operative and cutting procedures for the treatment of disease or injury, treatment of fractures and dislocations, and surgery required due to pregnancy, and all other obstetrical procedures." [8]

The auxiliary services often include anesthesia, diagnostic X-ray examinations, and laboratory services. Their scope is nearly always restricted by ceilings on the amount allowed.

The "surgical certificate" of the Michigan Medical Service, in force at the end of 1946, provided for surgical services rendered by the doctor of medicine in charge of the case; maternity care after the certificate has been in force nine consecutive months; diagnostic X-ray services not in excess of the value of $15; anesthesia services rendered by a doctor of medicine not in charge of the case, when in connection with services in the hospital; and emergency surgical services not requiring bed care, rendered in a regularly accredited hospital by a doctor of medicine during the first twenty-four hours following accidental injury.

Examples of plans providing for physicians' services other than surgical and obstetrical in case of hospitalization are the California Physicians' Service, the Iowa Medical Service, and the Marion County Medical Service, West Virginia.

The Massachusetts Medical Service covers surgical services in the home, physician's office, outpatient department, or inpatient department of a licensed general, maternity, or acute contagious disease hospital, up to twenty-one days per hospital admission or twenty-one days per illness or injury if the patient is not hospitalized; and "nonsurgical services of a general medical nature" for bed-patients in a licensed general, maternity, or acute contagious disease hospital up to twenty-one days per hospital admission.

Examples of organizations providing for nonsurgical service outside the hospital along with surgical and nonsurgical service for inpatients are the California Physicians' Service and the North Idaho District Medical Service Bureau.

Organization of professional and hospital services.—All plans operate on the principle of free choice. Usually they permit any duly licensed and registered physician to participate. The plan members may select any of the participating physicians in the area covered by the plan. In emergencies they may utilize the services of nonparticipating physicians.

The fee-for-service method of payment is generally employed. The rates are standardized through special fee schedules established by agreement between the medical societies and the plans. The Michigan Medical Service, for instance, in 1946 allowed from $10 to $50 for casts; $50 for removal of a breast tumor, internal hemorrhoidectomy, or hydrocele operation; $75 for an appendectomy, herniotomy, or compound fracture of the humerus; $100 for a myomectomy, Caesarean section, or gastrotomy; $125 for an ectopic pregnancy, radical mastoidectomy, or compound fracture of the femur; $150 for the extirpation of a rectal carcinoma, prostatectomy, or hysterectomy.

In a few states, such as California and Massachusetts, a modification of the fee-for-service system is in use. The items in the fee schedule are expressed in "units," and the value of each unit is determined by the total amount of money available for distribution. Nonparticipating physicians usually are allowed payments ranging from one half to the full amount paid to the participating physicians.

Hospital care is made available through definite arrangements with Blue Cross plans. Exceptions to this rule are few.

Prepayment rates.—The monthly prepayment rates, or "premiums," vary according to the scope of the service and the size of the family. In 1946, the rates for surgical service in the hospital ranged from $0.60 for one subscriber to $2.25 for subscribers and family dependents. Those for surgical and medical service were higher. The Iowa Medical Service, for instance, charged $1.25 for one subscriber and $3.25 for families taking the combined medical and surgical contract.

It must be borne in mind that these prepayments are in addition to those for hospitalization. The combined cost of the surgical and hospital service contracts vary from one state to the other.

In Michigan, in 1946, the monthly prepayment rates to be made by group subscribers to the surgical and hospital ward-service contract were $1.72 to $2.02, $4.20, and $4.85 for single persons, a family of two, and a family with dependent children, respectively. The corresponding figures for semiprivate service were $2.00 to $2.30, $4.70 and $5.35. In California, in 1947, the quarterly rates covering surgical and hospital service for members of the State Grange were $5.15 and $6.50 for male and female subscribers, respectively, $11.90 for a family of two, and $16.70 for a family of three. The annual rates were $18.60, $24.00, $45.60, and $64.80, respectively.

Administration.—All but a few plans are administered by special agencies created for this purpose and organized similarly. Boards of trustees (or directors), serving without remuneration, are responsible for the management of "the affairs, property and business" of the corporations. Their composition varies widely. In some instances, such as the North Dakota Physicians' Service and Surgical-Medical Care, Kansas City, Missouri, physicians are the only board members; in others they constitute the majority and nonmedical representatives the minority; and in still others, physicians have a relatively small number of seats.

In 1946, the board of trustees of the California Physicians' Service consisted of eleven physicians and four laymen; the

Blue Shield Plans

board of the Colorado Medical Service of twelve physicians and seven laymen, elected from and by the membership; and the board of the Massachusetts Medical Service of fifteen members, including five physicians and ten persons representing labor and management.

Often special committees are appointed by the boards. In Massachusetts, for instance, they include a "Central Professional Service Committee" to control and supervise the medical aspects of the plan and an "Actuarial Research Committee." In addition to boards and designated officers, there are paid executives and other administrative personnel for specific administrative tasks.

The Michigan Medical Service at the end of 1946 had a paid administrative staff that included five persons in the executive department, one medical director, five persons in the claims department, six "doctors relation representatives," and seventy clerical and other employees. In addition there were twenty persons assigned for the administration of services to veterans under a special contract with the Veterans Administration.

Recently medical society plans have tended to utilize the personnel of hospital service plans for certain administrative purposes. Although continuing as separate organizations, Blue Shield and Blue Cross plans have agreed on the coordination of some of their activities.

A pertinent example of extensive pooling of administrative personnel and costs is the agreement made in 1942 between the Massachusetts Hospital Service and the Massachusetts Medical Service. The Blue Cross plan undertakes to

(1) furnish office space for personnel serving both corporations; (2) supply services necessary for the acquisition of subscribers; (3) provide all administrative services, including billing, accounting and general operating supervision; (4) render bills on all outstanding Blue Shield memberships and use its best efforts to collect all such accounts receivable; (5) use efforts in the acquisition of

subscribers to Blue Shield similar in kind and degree to and consistent with its own acquisition policy, and consult with Blue Shield with respect to general program and detail.

Except for materials or services which are solely for the benefit of one of the corporations, charges are divided between the two plans in proportion to their subscriber incomes.[9] Under this arrangement the Massachusetts Medical Service at the end of 1946 had on its own full-time administrative staff only about thirty persons to audit and process claims.

The difficult problem of assuring maintenance of quality of service has been tackled by the Massachusetts Medical Service by the creation of "district professional service committees." They are expected from time to time to survey the quality of medical care rendered to subscribers in their districts, to report their findings to the "Central Professional Service Committee," and to investigate and report on disputes involving a participating physician's services to or conduct toward a subscriber.[10]

Approval.—Approval by the Council on Medical Service and Public Relations of the American Medical Association is given to those plans which conform with the requirements formulated by the Council. This approval carries with it the right to print the "seal of acceptance" on all official papers and in any promotional literature or display material.

The requirements set forth details as to local approval, professional control, arbitration, free choice of physician, patient-physician relationship, elements of successful operation, prepayment rates, type of benefits, content of subscriber contracts, promotional activities, enrollment practices, legal aspects, periodic reports, and re-examination of approval.[11]

Experience.—Dearth of published data precludes the presentation of an over-all picture of the experience of Blue Shield plans. The reports published up to the end of 1946 contain chiefly figures on financial operations and little, if any, information on the utilization of the programs. However, two statements are well substantiated. By far the greatest number of members come from the ranks of higher paid industrial workers and salaried employees in cities. The expenditures for acquisition and management usually exceed 10 per cent and often 15 per cent of the total premium income. In Massachusetts the operating expenses accounted for 39 per cent of subscriber income in 1943, 15.4 per cent in 1944, 14.1 per cent in 1945, and 14.8 per cent in 1946. In Michigan they constituted 20 per cent in 1940, about 15 per cent each in 1941 and 1942, 12 per cent in 1943, 11.4 per cent in 1944, 11.5 per cent in 1945, and 11.7 per cent in 1946.

Additional facts of general importance can be gleaned from a special study made by the Michigan Medical Service and from its annual reports. In the period from April 1, 1942, to March 31, 1944, the three most frequently rendered types of service were tonsillectomies (21.6 per cent), X-ray examinations (19 per cent), and deliveries (13.4 per cent). The three largest amounts paid out to the physicians were for gynecological operations (22.2 per cent), appendectomies (15.4 per cent), and deliveries (13.7 per cent). Female adults received approximately 46 per cent of all services, and the costs of their care accounted for slightly more than 58 per cent of all payments. Subscribers required 29 per cent of all services and 31 per cent of all payments, and family dependents received 71 per cent of all services at costs equal to 69 per cent of all payments. The total sums paid to the participating physicians amounted to $790,733 in 1941, $2,208,623 in 1942, $2,876,548 in 1943, $3,437,265 in 1944, $4,154,423 in 1945, and $5,106,280 in 1946.

Significant changes in basic policy had to be made by certain plans. The California Physicians' Service and the Michigan Medical Service originally offered complete physicians' service in the home, office, and hospital, but after a few years were forced to drop the "full coverage contracts." They found that the selection of risks was unfavorable, the demand for service much greater than anticipated, the cost far in excess of the premium income, and the amount of money available for payments to physicians so insufficient that prorating was the only resort immediately open. Compelled to choose between increase of the prepayment rates and curtailment of the benefits, the plans decided to limit the service, on the theory that the public demanded first of all protection against catastrophic illness.

Similar problems arose elsewhere. To solve them, some plans, such as Medical and Surgical Care, Inc. in Utica, New York, and Western New York Medical Plan, Inc. in Buffalo, New York, discontinued their original service programs and offered cash indemnity contracts only.

The response of the physicians in private practice to the plans varied from plan to plan. At the end of 1946, the proportion of eligible physicians actually participating in the services ranged from 40 per cent to nearly 100 per cent. It was 75 per cent in Michigan, 90 per cent in Massachusetts, and 83 per cent in California, the states with the largest enrollment in Blue Shield organizations.

Achievements.—The plans described before are manifestations of the medical profession's readiness to assume responsibility for the organization of medical service for self-supporting persons. They have tapped a keenly felt need and afforded the subscribers some degree of protection against a burdensome expense item. Exclusion of nonmedical practitioners from participation has created a monopoly for doctors of medicine and laid the foundation for the improvement of the quality of medical care.

The income of a considerable number of participating physicians has been increased through the stabilization of the purchasing power of the patients. Members of the medical profession who formerly have had no opportunity to familiarize themselves with the socioeconomic aspects of illness and of medicine have gained insight into the nature of the problem, the relative merits of the various approaches to its solution, and the administrative policies and procedures necessary to the successful operation of prepayment plans.

Shortcomings.—At present the plans are accessible only to persons enrolling in groups of a certain size and the vast majority exclusively to employed people and their family dependents. Thus many persons who can afford the prepayments are barred from enrollment. Limitations on income and age further reduce the number of eligible persons.

The exclusion of pre-existing conditions from service creates problems for the patients, the attending physicians, and the administrations. Limited in scope as they are, the programs meet only part of the medical care needs of the seriously sick and put many patients into the dilemma of making substantial additional expenditures for services not covered. They discourage the practice of preventive and psychosomatic medicine and place a premium on surgery. Reciprocity of service is practically nonexisting. The first step in this direction was taken in February, 1947, by the California Physicians' Service, which has suggested reciprocal agreements between nine plans in the western and southern states.

The Blue Shield plans can easily make arrangements for the payment of the services by the patients and the disbursement of funds to the physicians rendering care, but because of their method of organization have great difficulty in giving due consideration to the selection of competent physicians, the qualification of those rendering the services for which payment is claimed, and the supervision of the services performed as to indication and quality. Complicated intraprofessional problems are raised. Certain specialists are greatly benefited both professionally and financially—some receiving tens of thousands of dollars each and every year—while the general practitioners are relegated to a minor place in the program and have to be content with whatever is left in the family budget.

The policy of some plans to deny subscribers seat and voice

in the administration or to permit merely token representation of the public makes it hard to foster the sense of responsibility so important to the operation of an organized program and violates the principle of democratic control. Actually it has alienated many groups. The administrative cost is much too high, considering the very limited service that is to be managed. The maintenance of separate organizations for medical and hospital services emphasizes independence rather than interdependence, increases the overhead, and may easily lead to a situation where the two plans are working at cross-purposes.

SEVEN

Nonprofit Plans Covering Professional and Hospital Services: Individual Practice Plans

THE nonprofit prepayment plans which provide for a variety of services under the system of individual practice are alike in including hospitalization as well as the services of physicians in the home, office, and hospital but are dissimilar in their extent of coverage. Quite a few also cover certain dental services, some provide for drugs, and some for ambulance service. These "single-package plans," as they are called in promotional literature, usually employ the free-choice principle and the fee-for-service method of payment. Outstanding in this category are the plans organized by the medical societies in the states of Oregon and Washington and in the Territory of Hawaii, and the plans initiated by agencies of the United States Department of Agriculture. The first type will be reviewed but briefly, as detailed description would be repetitious. The second type will be analyzed in all its aspects because it affords an object lesson on the problems involved in voluntary medical care insurance for people in rural areas.

MEDICAL SOCIETY PLANS IN OREGON, WASHINGTON, AND HAWAII

The prepayment plans in the states of Oregon and Washington are in a class by themselves. Established by medical societies to meet the special needs of major industries of these states, they have evolved a pattern sharply contrasting to that of other medical society plans.

128   *Comprehensive Individual Practice Plans*

Pioneer plans were organized in Pierce County, Washington, in 1917, at Corvallis in Benton County, Oregon, in 1925, and at Salem, in Marion County, Oregon, in 1930. Medical societies in other counties followed suit. In Washington, in 1933, the Washington State Medical Bureau was set up for the purpose of coordinating and promoting the prepayment medical and hospital programs of its component members; at the end of 1946, twenty-three organizations were operating in the counties. In Oregon the development took a similar course. There the Oregon Physicians' Service was incorporated in 1941 to amalgamate antecedent local organizations. The total enrollment at the end of 1946 amounted to approximately 100,000 in Oregon and 260,000 in Washington.

In both states the prepayment plans strictly adhere to the principle of providing service rather than cash indemnity benefits, accept employed subscribers on the basis of group enrollment regardless of their earnings, and arrange for maintenance of membership of those who have left the original group. Most units also provide for family coverage. All plans offer professional services in the home, office, and hospital, together with hospitalization. Care by both general practitioners and specialists is available for periods ranging from six months to one year in the various counties. Hospitalization in wards, including all auxiliary services, is offered up to six months in most instances and longer in some; and provision of prescribed medicines and drugs and of ambulance service is part of most of the programs. Maternity care is included in the family contracts but not in the employee group contracts. In Oregon additional provisions are made for limited dental service, one complete physical examination a year, and prophylactic measures, such as smallpox vaccinations and inoculations.

The monthly prepayment rates charged by the Oregon Physicians' Service early in 1947 were $3.00 for one person

Comprehensive Individual Practice Plans 129

covered by the "employee group full coverage contract" and $2.00 for the unemployed spouse, $1.35 for the first child, $0.75 for the second child, and $0.50 for the third child covered by supplementary family contract. In Washington the monthly rates for the employed subscribers ranged from $2.00 to $3.75, the greatest number of contracts being available at $2.50. The rates for families of three or more persons ranged from $5.25 to $10.50 per month.

The vast majority of all physicians in active practice in these states are participating in the prepayment plans. At the end of 1946, the proportions were approximately 95 per cent in Oregon and about 85 per cent in Washington.

Both organizations are approved by the Council on Medical Service and Public Relations of the American Medical Association and administered by boards of directors composed entirely of physicians. Noteworthy is their comparatively low overhead. In recent years it was between 7 and 9 per cent in Washington and in the neighborhood of 10 per cent in Oregon. In Oregon less than 10 per cent of the persons covered by the prepayment plans required expenditures of more than $100 for doctor and hospital bills in any one year, and the cost of their care absorbed about 30 per cent of the total expenditures.[1] In Washington about 60 per cent of the total service payments in 1946 were made to physicians.

The Hawaii Medical Service Association, endorsed by the Honolulu County Medical Society, was founded in 1938 and had grown to an organization with 18,800 participants by the end of 1946. In contrast to the plans in Oregon and Washington, it has set an income limit for eligibility, restricting enrollment to persons earning less than $6,000 per year. Its services include hospitalization in wards as well as home, office, and hospital care by physicians for surgical conditions and a limited number of home and office visits for nonsurgical conditions.

PLANS FOR LOW-INCOME FARM FAMILIES

History and trends of development.—In 1936, the Resettlement Administration of the United States Department of Agriculture, later the Farm Security Administration (F.S.A.), initiated voluntary prepayment plans for medical care as part of a general rehabilitation program for low-income farmers unable to secure credit from commercial sources. This policy was motivated by the conviction that a family in good health was a better credit risk than a family in bad health.[2]

The number of counties served by such plans grew rapidly from eight in 1936 to a peak of 1,120 in 1943, but declined to 1,048 in 1945 and 951 in 1946. Originally, almost all units were limited geographically to one county each, and district organization was the exception. Later a tendency appeared to establish multi-county or state-wide organizations. There were 1,014 units in 1,074 counties at the end of the fiscal year 1941–42. In contrast, only 743 units were serving 1,048 counties at the end of the fiscal year 1944–45, and 635 units were serving 951 counties at the end of the fiscal year 1945–46.

The number of families covered rose from less than 1,000 in 1936 to a maximum of 117,616 with 616,465 persons in August, 1942, and decreased sharply in subsequent years. The 743 units in operation at the end of June, 1945, had a total enrollment of 55,525 families, comprising 283,100 persons.

With the passage of the Farmers Home Administration Act of August 14, 1946, and the abolition of the Farm Security Administration, an entirely new situation has arisen. The field personnel of this agency is authorized to encourage borrowers to use part of their loans to pay for membership in existing health service plans but is enjoined from organizing, conducting, or managing group prepayment plans. As the curtain has fallen over the F.S.A. plans of the past, the final account of this experiment can now be presented.

Eligibility requirements.—In general, the plans accepted only persons who were borrowers of the F.S.A. and extended eligibility to the whole family rather than the breadwinner only. The word "family" was commonly interpreted as meaning the farmer and "those individuals in his immediate family and other persons of his household residing with and dependent upon him for support." In many instances the farmers were permitted to continue their membership after having paid off their loans from the F.S.A. About one fourth of the plans accepted low-income farm families who were not clients of the F.S.A. This tendency was most pronounced in the western states.

Type of illness covered.—The plans usually provided services required for treatment of acute illness (including acute surgical conditions) and for prenatal, obstetrical and postnatal care. With a few notable exceptions they were organized "for the purpose of furnishing emergency medical care," although in actual practice they provided for most of the services of physicians, especially those of general practitioners, without regard to their emergency nature. A liberal declaration of policy appeared in the following model form prepared by the Region VII office of the F.S.A.:

"Emergency" shall be deemed to refer only to such medical care as is necessary in treating acute illnesses or acute recurrences of chronic conditions of such nature as to cause actual suffering, interfering with earning capacity, endangering life, or threatening some permanent new handicap as is preventable when medical care is sought . . .

Type and scope of service.—All the plans offered one or more of the following services: general physicians', surgeons', dentists', hospitalization, and supply of some drugs. Medical service in the home of the patient and the office of the physician was always available, and service in the hospital was often included in the scope of programs covering physicians' care. Hospitalization was usually provided in wards. It included board and room, general nursing care, use of the operating and delivery rooms, certain clinical laboratory services, X-ray examinations, anesthetics, dressings, and routine drugs. As a rule, it was restricted to a certain number of days per year or cases of illness. Drugs, if provided, were either those ordinarily furnished by the physician himself or those listed in one of the official formularies. Not infrequently, dental care and hospitalization were organized under separate programs.

The scope, combination, and extent of these services varied widely from unit to unit and from one part of the country to the other. The following figures for the fiscal years 1941–42 and 1944–45 will serve to show not only the general patterns that have emerged but the changes that have taken place.

At the end of the fiscal year 1941–42, there were 787 units offering physicians' service alone or in combination with other services, 221 units offering dental services only, and six units offering hospitalization alone or together with surgical service. At the end of the fiscal year 1944–45, there were 469 units offering physicians' service alone or in combination with other services, 233 units offering dental service only, and 41 units offering hospital or surgical service or a combination of these services.

Of 117,460 families enrolled in health service units at the end of the fiscal year 1942, when membership was at a record high, 92.8 per cent were eligible for general physicians' service, 60.2 per cent for surgical service, 54.8 per cent for hospitalization, 39.8 per cent for drug service, and 41.7 per cent for dental care. At that time the emphasis was on provision of general practitioners' service; surgical care ranked second, hospitalization third, and drugs were made available to about 40 per cent of the families.

In the fiscal year 1944–45, the picture was quite different, reflecting the war-created shortage of physicians in rural areas and the increased popularity of hospitalization programs. Hospitalization had come to occupy a dominant place, being available to nearly three fourths of all families, and general practitioners' service as well as drug service had sharply declined in relative frequency. Of all families enrolled on June 30, 1945, 74 per cent were eligible for hospital service, 61.6 per cent for surgical service, 61.3 per cent for general physicians' service, 28.9 per cent for dental service, and 21 per cent for drugs.

Organization of professional and hospital services.—A "working understanding" with each state medical society has been considered by the F.S.A. a prerequisite to the development of local plans. Under the general terms of the state agreement, the local plans were worked out with county medical societies.

Participation in the local plans was open to all duly licensed physicians and dentists residing in the respective areas. The members of the plans had free choice among the physicians and dentists who were party to the local agreements.

Payment for professional services was made primarily through the fee-for-service system. The fees were set by the local professional groups. They were uniform for all participating physicians and dentists in a given area but differed widely from county to county. In general they were either identical with or slightly below those ordinarily charged in local private practice. The bills of physicians and dentists were settled monthly or, occasionally, quarterly, and the amount paid out depended upon the funds earmarked and available for distribution in a given period.

In response to the wishes of the professional societies in their areas, a small number of plans had adopted the "capitation" method of payment, allotting to the participating physicians a fixed amount according to the number of families on their lists. As of June 30, 1945, the capitation system was used by 74 units offering physicians' service, 10 units offering dental service, and 9 units offering hospital service. The salary method was employed by some dental plans.

Hospitalization was made available through contracts with facilities in the area of each unit. The participating hospitals usually received payment according to the number of patient days rendered, at prevailing rates for ward service.

Organization of payment.—The Farm Security Administration advanced funds in the form of loans to farmers qualifying for aid. These loans were for the purpose of purchasing seed, feed, fertilizer, and farm and house equipment, as well as for family subsistence. Part of them could be used to cover the cost of the medical care program. As a general rule, those joining a plan agreed to make regular annual prepayments toward the cost of the service.

Annual prepayment was universal because of the special conditions governing the operation of F.S.A. plans. The rates were determined locally and established on a family basis. Their size depended on the type of the program, the scope of service covered, the financial resources of the borrowers, and, often, the size of the family. In 1945, the units offering medical, surgical, hospital, and dental services usually charged membership fees ranging from $30 to $50 per year; units offering only hospital service charged rates ranging from $10 to $18; and dental care plans cost $4 to $7. In a few instances the rates differed from this norm.

Administration.—The Farm Security Administration had a "health services division" that was responsible to the Administrator for the formulation of the broad policies in regard to the organization of plans and for the guidance and general supervision of the units. It utilized regional offices, some of which were staffed with medical officers and nearly all with "health service specialists," to carry out such administrative functions as could be decentralized.

Authority for management of the local units was given to private persons, the trustees, or to nonprofit associations rather than to governmental agencies.

The trustees were responsible for holding the funds of the

Comprehensive Individual Practice Plans 135

unit and paying the professional persons and hospitals. In most instances they were chosen by the F.S.A. County Supervisors in consultation with representatives of the participating professional groups and the plan members. Very often they were appointed because of their interest in the plans and their business experience, without being members of the organizations, and received some financial compensation for the time spent on the management of the funds. Questions arising in the course of the operation of the program were handled by the trustee either alone or in consultation with the F.S.A. County Supervisor and representatives of the enrolled farmers. At the end of 1946 the trusteeship system was being utilized by more than half of all units. In a few instances, committees of members had been formed to assist the trustees, the professional groups, and the F.S.A. people in settling questions of policy and operation.

Possibly as many as one fourth of the units, mostly in the western states, had developed formal associations with elected boards of directors and officers to take full responsibility for all aspects of administration. The members of the plans, or all F.S.A. borrowers, usually had a voice in selecting those who were to conduct the affairs of the associations. The boards included representatives of the participating farmers as a rule and representatives of the participating physicians occasionally.

Regardless of the method of administrative organization, the physicians and dentists serving under the programs had full authority over all professional matters. Their administrative duties and powers included the reviewing and auditing of bills submitted and—to a slight extent—the control of the professional behavior of the participating members of the professions. To discharge these functions, the local medical and dental societies usually appointed special committees ("reviewing" or "auditing" committees), with one physician, or dentist in the case of dental service, acting as chairman and other representatives serving in rotation. A few plans offering hospitalization had their affairs handled by the Blue Cross plans operating in their areas.

The Farmers Home Administration Act of August 14, 1946, deprived the units of the active help of the field personnel employed by that agency and thus eliminated one of the most important sources of administrative council and guidance.

Experience.—More than ten years of experience have produced a large body of information on both the merits of the basic policies and the utilization of the programs. Pertinent statistical data have been published regularly by the F.S.A.[3] The outstanding facts will be summarized here.

In the fiscal year 1940-41, about 60 per cent of all eligible families in counties with physicians' service plans were enrolled in such units. Subsequently the figures declined constantly—to 55 per cent in 1941-42, 49 per cent in 1942-43, 41 per cent in 1943-44, and 30.8 per cent as of June 30, 1945. In that year, 12.2 per cent of all eligible F.S.A. borrowers were enrolled for physicians' service and surgical service, 14.6 per cent for hospitalization, and 5.8 per cent for dental care. Participation in general and membership in specific types of plans varied greatly from region to region, from state to state within the same region, and from unit to unit within the same state.

The turnover has been heavy, and only a small percentage of all members have continued their membership over several years. About one fourth of those who at the end of the fiscal year 1942-43 were enrolled in units offering physicians' services or dental care were still holding membership at the end of the fiscal year 1944-45. The percentage of persons covered by hospital service plans was somewhat higher, coming close to one third. One of the major reasons for the turnover was the loss of eligibility after the families had become self-supporting with repayment of their loans. Another was dissatisfaction with the plans on the part of the farmers, physicians, or both.

Comprehensive Individual Practice Plans 137

There is some indication that the families who stayed in the plans were primarily those requiring much service.

With few exceptions the members of the health professions and the hospitals had been willing to give the plans a fair trial and cooperated, some wholeheartedly and some reluctantly. At the end of the fiscal year 1944–45, the lists of participants contained the names of 68 per cent of the licensed physicians in active practice in the areas covered by the plans, of 65 per cent of the eligible dentists, and of 76 per cent of the hospitals in the respective districts. In some states 100 per cent participation was recorded.

The number of physicians' calls (office, home, and hospital) per 1,000 eligible persons in a number of reporting units was 1,344 in 1942–43, 1,320 in 1943–44, and 1,322 in 1944–45. The great majority of these services were office calls. The rate of 1,322 physicians' calls reported for 1944–45 included 1,071 office calls, 207 home calls, and 44 hospital calls per 1,000 eligible persons. In 1940–41, in regions I, III, V, and VII, there were recorded 2.70, 6.54, 2.92, and 9.49 office calls, respectively, for every home call.[4]

A detailed study of the experience of F.S.A. plans in five counties of Ohio during the period 1940–43 showed 200 contacts with physicians per 100 male persons and 289 contacts per 100 female persons in the course of a year. The rates for females exceeded those for males in every age group. More than half of all calls were for treatment of diseases of the respiratory, digestive, and genito-urinary systems. Nearly one third of the physicians' calls made for women of childbearing age were for illnesses and conditions related to pregnancy, childbirth, and their complications.[5]

Figures on the frequency of hospitalization are not available. The number of hospital days per 1,000 eligible persons was 188 in 1941–42, 228 in 1942–43, 199 in 1943–44, 294–295 in 1944–45, and 368 in 1945–46, with very pronounced variations by states.

138 *Comprehensive Individual Practice Plans*

Year in and year out, all but a few F.S.A. plans had to wrestle with the problem of meeting their obligations, as the approved bills of physicians, dentists, and hospitals exceeded the available funds. Consequently, prorating has been the rule and full payment the exception. The principle of scaling down was applied in different ways. Either all bills were prorated uniformly or charges for certain services were given preference. Where different funds for the various types of service were set up, the bills often were cut to quite different degrees. What the physicians, dentists, druggists, and hospitals finally received was a product of two processes, approval and reconciliation; at best it was what they had claimed and at worst it was a disappointingly small fraction of their claims.

In the fiscal year 1940–41, the units offering physicians' service alone or a combination of various services paid the following percentages of the approved charges: physicians and surgeons, 60.7 per cent (with a range by regions from 41.7 per cent to 74.3 per cent); hospitals, 74.2 per cent (47.3 per cent to 97.7 per cent); druggists 78.9 per cent (50 per cent to 100 per cent); and dentists, 80.5 per cent (72 per cent to 97.7 per cent). Units offering only dental service paid an average of 83.1 per cent of the approved charges. In the fiscal year 1944–45 the situation was better. Of the approved charges, physicians and surgeons received 80 per cent under plans covering both types and surgeons 86.3 per cent under plans confined to surgical service; hospitals, 87 per cent; druggists, 85 per cent; and dentists, 92.3 per cent.

The total payments for all types of service in 1944–45 amounted to approximately one and a quarter million dollars. Of this sum, more than two thirds were for the services of physicians, more than one fifth for hospital care, and the remainder for dental services and drugs.

Achievements.—By fostering voluntary cooperation between the physicians, dentists, druggists, and hospitals on the one hand and the borrowers of the F.S.A. on the other, a

Comprehensive Individual Practice Plans 139

governmental agency has met on common ground with the private professions and voluntary hospitals. All have worked together, each in its rightful place. This is an achievement of the first order.

The medical care programs began as a side line of a depression-born, tax-supported rehabilitation program for certain groups of farmers. By their large number, wide geographic dispersion, and substantial membership, they came to play an important role in rural health activities during the late thirties and early forties. This is all the more important as in the past farmers have been the stepchildren of health service.

The rural people, so often called "the most individualistic and independent-minded part of the entire population," have learned to appreciate the financial and psychological advantages that can be derived from pooling available resources for protection against the economic burden of illness. They have discovered the significance of organized self-help through group prepayment for health service and have obtained some measure of security. All were financially assisted in budgeting for their basic medical care expenditures and enabled to see the physician oftener and earlier, before their condition had become critical. Many received more service at low cost than they would have otherwise been able to procure. Not a few experienced regular medical care for the first time in their lives. All these facts combined to create a public opinion overwhelmingly favorable to the plans.

The participating physicians, dentists, druggists, and hospitals benefited from the plans, although to a widely varying extent. In some instances, members of the health professions were enabled to settle or to hold regular office hours in places where practice had not been attractive at all. Many physicians and dentists established, or strengthened, their relationship with the patients, derived additional income from a group of people hitherto unable to make regular expenditures for medical care, and saved time and money for collection of charges. The physicians found practice less strenuous, because the patients grew accustomed to coming to the office early rather than requesting home visits after the condition had become serious. On the whole, the total collections of the participating physicians compared favorably with those in earlier years when there was no F.S.A. medical program. The farmers for whom the plans were organized never had spent much on medical care. If they were badly in need of service, they had tried to pay, but often found it impossible to foot the bill within a reasonable period of time, if at all. The experience of several physicians in rural areas of a midwestern state reveals that during the period from 1930 to 1940 the collections from farmers not covered by a program averaged about 70 per cent of the charges, with a low of 50 per cent and a high of 83 per cent. Many other physicians in rural areas had never been able to collect much more than 60 to 70 per cent in practices wherein only a small fraction of patients were farmers of the class which later became eligible for F.S.A. plans. A case in point is the story of a physician in Ohio. Prior to the establishment of the F.S.A. plan he had rendered service to thirty-six families and collected $150 out of a total of $900 charged. If these families had been in a group plan at that time, he would have received about $700 at the rate of payment prevailing in 1942.[6] The hospitals too were benefited by the payments for care rendered to F.S.A. plan members. The income from this source made it easier for many a rural hospital to meet its operating costs. The possibility of obtaining the services of physicians and hospitals improved maternity care, as the farmers were no longer dependent on the untrained midwives.

Utilization of the services provided by the local and state health departments, the state agencies in charge of vocational rehabilitation, and other health and welfare agencies was encouraged and, in many instances, organized by the F.S.A. personnel, with the result that some coordination between the prepayment plans and other programs was achieved and the service to the farmers improved.

The farmers, the professional persons, and the employees of the F.S.A. learned by trial and error the essential factors governing medical care insurance. They all were stimulated to do much thinking about ways and means of improving rural health services by planning.

Shortcomings.—The F.S.A. plans showed all the limitations of voluntary medical care insurance to a much larger degree than observed in general. In addition, they suffered from weaknesses that resulted from the policies and procedures followed in initiation and operation. These shortcomings were freely admitted by all who had firsthand knowledge of the programs. The Farm Security Administration and its subdivisions, the borrowers, the members of the health professions, and the hospitals realized that the medical care programs were nothing but a stopgap, the only expedient that could be used under the conditions prevailing in rural areas.

The F.S.A. plans were designed to provide emergency service for persons with "thin pocketbooks" and high incidence of sickness and injury. They served families living on isolated farms or, at best, some miles from a village or small town in areas lacking most of the basic public health services. Any voluntary prepayment plan established under such circumstances bears within it the seed of its own death. It is not by accident that many units were forced to terminate operation after a short period of trial or could barely manage to struggle along. The factors responsible for this situation were the limitation of coverage to an economically weak group with many poor risks; the relatively small number of borrowers living in many of the counties, a fact that militated against any attempt to spread the risks and share the costs on a sound actuarial basis; the amount of service required for treatment of acute illnesses, serious accidents, exacerbations of neglected conditions, and diseases incurred because of the absence of even the rudimentary machinery for mass prevention; and the heavy turnover of membership that accentuated the adverse selection of risks.

The limitations on the type, scope, amount, and period of service were dictated by necessity. Many of the F.S.A. borrowers could hardly afford even the modest contributions necessary for the support of a very limited service, and too few could make the regular prepayments needed for a more inclusive plan. There was much enthusiasm but too little money to spend on health services. Small wonder that the amount of care received by the members of the plans, although larger than before, remained far below standards of quantitative adequacy. Preventive medicine has been conspicuous by its absence.

The problem of improving the quality of service proved to be impossible of solution for most of the F.S.A. plans except the dental care programs carried out by trailer service. In many areas competent general practitioners were few, specialists lacking, diagnostic facilities scarce and far away, and hospitals absent, distant, or of low standard. By force of circumstances, the F.S.A. plans had to accept hospital facilities and professional personnel pretty much as they were before the organization of the programs. All they could do was to offer a payment plan for the readily available services and—much against their own conviction—side-step efforts to raise the standards of medical care. Many farmers would have paid higher rates and a larger number would have joined, if they had been sure of getting real value for their money. "Can the professional groups deliver the goods?"—this was the question raised again and again by many thoughtful farmers as well as all the F.S.A. personnel concerned.

The scaling down of the approved charges of physicians, dentists, druggists, and hospitals could not fail to impair the reputation of the plans. Moderate prorating produced the impression that "charity prices" were paid and discouraged good service. As one physician remarked, "I do not mind chatting with a patient for 60 cents but I simply cannot afford giving him a real examination for this fee." Heavy cuts, particularly if coming on top of reductions made in the process of approval, caused strong resentment among the members of the professions and, in a number of instances, turned ardent proponents of a plan into bitter opponents. Those who agree to render services under a prepayment program are entitled to a fair return for their work. If they are disappointed in their expectations and continuously must feel the keen edge of the axe of prorating, they will inevitably—and justifiably—state their dissatisfaction in unmistakable language and may ultimately decide to refuse further participation in the service. A grudge based on a bad experience in the past may well result in distrust of any proposal advanced by a governmental agency in the future.

The trusteeship system of management proved to be utterly inadequate. For all practical purposes it was an organization resembling a primitive bank establishment in charge of the money with which the farmer paid his doctor, dentist, druggist, and hospital. It was not suited to the performance of administrative functions and it could do little, if anything, to develop leadership and initiative among the members of the plans. It succeeded in some areas only because the F.S.A. personnel, an exceptionally interested physician, or a community leader gave freely of their time and energy.

The creation of formal associations was beset with difficulties because leadership was hard to find among the group of farmers eligible for enrollment. Their administration was anything but easy because of the reluctance of the individual members to take active part in the management.

Critics of the F.S.A. plans have been answered with the arguments that a meager proposition is better than none and that initiation of a limited program provides a starting point for gradual development. Actually, the hope for marked improvement never materialized, although the participating physicians, dentists, druggists, and hospitals as well as the plan members in various areas repeatedly and earnestly urged the substitution of an adequate program of medical care for a makeshift solution resembling a glorified relief service.

EXPERIMENTAL RURAL HEALTH PROGRAMS

In 1942, the Interbureau Committee on Post-War Programs of the United States Department of Agriculture initiated voluntary "experimental health programs" in seven counties for all persons securing most of their income "from agricultural pursuits" or for all residents of rural areas rather than for borrowers of the F.S.A. only. These plans were organized to determine whether the deficiencies of the F.S.A. plans could be eliminated and comprehensive medical care could be provided by accepting all farm families regardless of income, basing the prepayments on ability to pay, and allotting substantial subsidies from tax funds.

The authority to grant federal funds was terminated by the Farmers Home Administration Act of August 14, 1946. Thus the plans received a stunning blow.

The programs provided for the services of general practitioners, specialists, dentists, and hospitals. Some also included drug service and home nursing.

The Rural Health Services Association in Newton County, Mississippi, in 1945, made services available in case of sickness, accident and maternity. The program included physicians' services, dental care, hospitalization, and special diagnostic and therapeutic procedures. It excluded "conditions not curable or for which institutional care is provided and available," prescribed drugs, eyeglasses, surgical and orthopedic appliances, and dentures. The "practitioner services," interpreted as services ordinarily rendered by the family doctor, included office, home, and hospital calls; ordinary medical, minor surgical, prenatal, obstetrical, and postnatal care;

Comprehensive Individual Practice Plans 145

medicines and drugs ordinarily dispensed or used; annual health examinations; venereal disease treatment where not provided by the public health department; routine laboratory tests of urine and blood; and consultations. "Specialists' services" included all major surgical operations necessary "to preserve life or limb and materially improve the health of the patient." Dentists' services included extractions, relief of pain, and eradication of infection when necessary in the judgment of the dentist to protect the general health, and amalgam alloy or synthetic porcelain fillings where necessary to eradicate infection or preserve the teeth. Hospitalization was provided for a period up to fourteen days per family and year. Special procedures available "within reasonable limits" included X-ray examinations, basic metabolism tests, electrocardiograms, oxygen therapy, blood transfusions, and X-ray and radium treatments.

In general, the organization of the experimental health programs was based on the pattern chosen for the F.S.A. plans. The operating costs were met by prepayments of the participating families, with contributions set at 6 per cent of the annual net cash income of the family, and by tax funds allotted by the federal government in amounts bringing the total annual prepayments into the pool to a sum averaging about $50 per participating family. The administrative responsibility was vested in local nonprofit corporations.

The experience of these programs is important for two reasons. Service was offered to people in rural areas regardless of income, and the prepayment rates were placed on the basis of ability to pay rather than on fixed amounts derived from purely actuarial facts.[7] In the first year of operation, 9,287 families with 41,700 persons were enrolled in seven plans. By 1943–44, enrollment had declined to 6,663 families with 31,833 persons in six plans. By the end of 1946, approximately 6,700 families with about 28,950 persons were enrolled in three plans.

The membership at the end of the fiscal years 1942–43 and

1943–44 represented 49.7 and 45.1 per cent, respectively, of the farm population in the areas served by the plans. At the end of the fiscal year 1945–46, the corresponding figure was 49.6 per cent. The average annual prepayment actually made by the participating families were $10.16 in 1942–43, $19.38 in 1943–44, $19.37 in 1944–45, and $27.80 in 1945–46. The tax subsidy allotted by the Federal government amounted to $40.31 per family in 1942–43, $28.79 in 1943–44, $29.65 in 1944–45, and $34.52 in 1945–46. These funds constituted 81, 62, 60, and 55 per cent, respectively, of the operating costs in these years. The approved charges of those rendering service in 1942–43 were paid at the rate of 55.9 per cent for general practitioners' services, 67 per cent for surgical service, 97.4 per cent for dental service, 88 per cent for hospitalization, and 87.6 per cent for drug service. In the fiscal year 1945–46, the percentage of approved charges paid were 59 per cent for physicians' services, 59.9 per cent for surgical service, 91.3 per cent for dental service, 73.5 per cent for hospitalization, and 95.1 per cent for drug service.

The number of services per 1,000 eligible persons per year was:

	1942–43	1945–46
Physicians' services		
Cases	1,408	1,431
Calls	2,917	3,208
Surgical services		
Cases	70.4	62.6
Tonsillectomies	34.3	14.3
Appendectomies	8.4	7.4
Gynecological operations	9.0	7.0
Dental services		
Cases	294	298
Extractions	571	467
Fillings	368	383
Hospitalization		
Admissions	110	113
Days of care	424	611

With the inclusion of obstetrical service in the plans, the role of the untrained midwives has been reduced to insignificance. Telling is the experience of the plan in Cass County, Texas, which began operation in 1942. There the proportion of all births attended by a physician rose from 65.3 per cent in 1938 to 78.4 per cent in 1944 and that of negro births attended by a physician from 6 per cent in 1938 to 41.4 per cent in 1944. In 1938, only 4.7 per cent of all births occurred in hospitals, and all of them were in the white population. By 1944, the percentage of hospital births had reached 43.3 for all groups, 59.3 for the white population, and 12.8 for the negroes. The increase in the proportion of hospital births substantially exceeded the increase observed in adjacent counties without prepayment plans.

The experimental health programs have achieved more than the F.S.A. plans. Assisted in their development by elimination of economic restrictions on eligibility, they could reach broader groups of the population. Aided by heavy subsidies from federal funds they could provide for more comprehensive service. But they suffered the same difficulties and showed essentially the same weaknesses as the F.S.A. plans. The experiences of both types support the conclusion that local voluntary prepayment plans for farmers are not suited to the attainment of complete coverage of the rural population and adequacy of medical care. This has been fully realized by the Secretary of Agriculture [8] and all those who have watched the experiments closely.

EIGHT

Group Practice Plans

History and trends of development.—Prepayment plans for medical care operated on the basis of group practice were organized relatively early under various auspices.

Industrial plans were the first to utilize this system. Some of them were developed and administered by the companies. Others were set up by the workers in the form of employees' mutual aid associations and to a varying degree were financially and administratively assisted by the employers. Examples are the Northern Pacific Beneficial Association, Northern Pacific Railway Company, St. Paul, Minnesota, founded in 1882; the Consolidated Edison Employees' Mutual Aid Society, New York City, incorporated in 1906; the plan of the Tennessee Coal, Iron and Railroad Company, Fairfield, Alabama, established in 1913; the Stanocola Employees' Medical and Hospital Association, Baton Rouge, Louisiana, founded in 1924; the Gates Mutual Benefit Club, Denver, Colorado, organized in 1929; the programs developed by the Tennessee Valley Authority at various construction projects, the first being instituted at Norris Dam in 1933;[1] and the health plans at the Kaiser industries, in particular the Permanente Foundation Health Plan, Oakland, California, and the Northern Permanente Foundation, Vancouver, Washington, which were organized in 1942.[2]

A second category of group practice prepayment plans owed its origin to the initiative of people forming cooperatives outside industry. These plans, organized for the purpose of securing medical care for association members and their families, observed all the principles of cooperation in formulating their programs, educating their members, providing for facilities of their own, organizing the professional staffs, and administering the services.[3] Examples of consumer cooperatives owning and administering prepayment plans for medical care in predominantly rural areas are the Farmers' Union Hospital Association, Elk City, Oklahoma, (1929); the South Plains Cooperative Hospital Association at Amherst, Texas (1941); the Northwest Community Hospital Association at Mooreland, Oklahoma (1941); and the Achenbach Memorial Hospital Association at Hardtner, Kansas (1941). Among the cooperatives serving people in urban areas are the Group Health Association, Washington, D.C. (1937); the Community Health Center, Two Harbors, Minnesota (1944); the Labor Health Institute, St. Louis, Missouri (1945); and the Group Health Co-Operative of Puget Sound, Seattle, Washington (1946). In the years 1946 and 1947 consumer cooperatives spread westward from the Mississippi River, especially in Texas. To guide and coordinate this movement a national organization, the Cooperative Health Federation of America, was founded in 1946.

Groups of physicians in private practice organized in partnership form were responsible for the development of the third type of prepayment plans—those initiated, owned, and administered by physicians. Among the pioneers were the Ross-Loos Medical Group, Los Angeles, California (1929); the Trinity Hospital, Little Rock, Arkansas (1931); and the Milwaukee Medical Center, Milwaukee, Wisconsin (1936).

The first large-scale attempt to develop a community-wide group practice prepayment plan sponsored and directed by community representatives was made in New York City. There the Health Insurance Plan of Greater New York was incorporated in 1944 and began operation early in 1947.

The total number of group practice prepayment plans and their membership cannot be given at present, as the definition of group practice is debated and the published reports include group practice plans financed entirely out of company resources or tax funds without application of the insurance principle. A special study undertaken by the United States Public Health Service in 1946 showed that 56 of 368 group practice organizations with three or more full-time physicians were offering prepayment plans. These groups were located primarily in large communities of the Pacific, Mountain, and South Atlantic states. There were none in the New England states.[4]

Closely related to the group practice prepayment plans described in this chapter are some of the student health services at institutions of higher learning. These furnish complete medical care as a part of the privileges covered by the tuition fees and utilize the method of group practice. The outstanding example is the program at the University of Michigan, which dates back to 1913.

Legal aspects.—Establishment and operation of group practice prepayment plans is subject to state laws. These laws vary greatly from one state to another and differ according to the auspices and form of organization of the programs.

Business concerns may initiate and maintain group practice prepayment plans for their employees, as the powers specifically granted in their certificates of incorporation include acts designed to protect and aid the employees. According to court interpretation, the reasonable care of its employees is a duty resting upon the corporation, and the proper discharge of that duty is merely transacting the business of the corporation.

Nonprofit organizations incorporated under state regulatory laws may make agreements with duly licensed physicians to furnish service to their members. In such cases the physicians are in a position legally known as that of "independent contractors." Their professional responsibility and independence are maintained and safeguarded by specific provisions that usually are set forth in bylaws. Recent legislation in the states of New York and Washington has created a firm legal basis for such agreements. The New York law, passed in 1947, permits a corporation organized under Article IX–C of the Insurance Law to employ duly licensed physicians or to enter into "contracts with duly licensed physicians or with partnerships or groups of duly licensed physicians to practice medicine on its behalf for persons insured under its contracts or policies."[5] The Washington law, adopted in 1947, authorizes prepayment agreements with "any corporation, cooperative group or association, doctor, or group of doctors." In contrast to many other states, it permits professional and hospital services to be covered through one plan by defining "health care services" as "medical, surgical, hospital and other therapeutic services."[6]

In a number of states it is questionable whether and under what conditions duly licensed physicians in private practice may lawfully practice their profession as groups in the form of a copartnership or an "unincorporated association" and pool the funds received. To remove any lingering doubt, the state of New York in 1947 passed legislation permitting physicians to practice medicine as partners or in groups and to pool fees and monies received, either by the partnerships or groups or by the individual members thereof, for professional services furnished by any individual physician, member, or employee of such partnership or group or to share, divide, or apportion the fees and monies received by them or by the partnership or group in accordance with a partnership or other agreement.[7]

A formidable barrier to the development of group practice prepayment plans has been created in some states by recent legislation governing nonprofit medical care corporations. In several states, such as Michigan and Illinois, the laws stipulate that every duly licensed and registered physician shall have the right to register with the corporation for service. Unless developed in every part of the respective states, group practice organizations could not qualify for incorporation, as they can admit only a certain number of all physicians practicing in their area. In other states, such as New Jersey, New Hampshire, and Tennessee, participation of the majority of all eligible physicians in the area of the plans is required to make establishment and operation lawful, and thus, at present, the door is closed to experimentation with group practice prepayment plans.

Eligibility requirements.—Group enrollment of employed persons is emphasized, but many plans permit individual enrollment of any applicant at slightly higher rates under certain conditions and provide for continuation of subscription on an individual basis for members who originally joined under group contracts.

The majority of plans set age limits for new members, and some require initial medical examination of individual subscribers, applicants who have had "chronic or recurring" conditions in the past, older persons, or family dependents. Nearly all accept subscribers regardless of their earnings, and the relatively few which do use income as yardstick of eligibility follow a liberal policy.

Family dependents as well as breadwinners are enrolled by most of the plans outside industry and by some of those in industry. Not infrequently, they must meet special requirements for admission or pay extra charges for specified services. In some instances they are eligible for selected services only.

Type of illness covered.—As a general rule the services of the prepayment plans are available for treatment of diseases and injuries not covered by Workmen's Compensation acts or other laws. Exclusions are few and apply primarily to prolonged treatment of patients with mental disease or tuberculosis, to drug addiction and alcoholism, to certain types of service, such as cosmetic surgery, and to pre-existing conditions. Maternity care is an integral part of almost all the programs.

Many of the organizations in industry are designed to provide care for occupational injuries and diseases as well as for nonoccupational conditions. In such cases the companies pay

Group Practice Plans

for services rendered under Workmen's Compensation laws.

Type and scope of service.—Inclusion of preventive as well as curative services and broad scope of the programs are the characteristic features of the group practice prepayment plans.

The great majority of the organizations provide for the services of physicians, specialists as well as general practitioners, at the home of the patient, the clinic, and the hospital; clinical laboratory tests; diagnostic and therapeutic X-ray services; physiotherapy; and hospitalization, including all ancillary services. Many cover such preventive measures as regular physical examinations, dental examinations, immunizations, and vaccinations. Some include limited dental treatment, visiting nurse service, specified drugs and appliances prescribed for nonhospitalized patients, radium therapy, and ambulance service, and a few have recently added organized health education, medical social service, and nutrition departments.

A relatively small number of the plans are limited to professional services but do make arrangements for hospitalization at fixed rates and for the purchase of drugs and selected appliances, such as eyeglasses, at discount.

Organization of professional services.—The plans operate either from their own clinics, located in functional buildings or occupying rented space in commercial buildings, or from hospitals of their own. The clinic facilities include well-equipped clinical and roentgenological laboratories, often also pharmacies and physiotherapy divisions, and occasionally additional departments, such as optical shops. There is always provision for twenty-four hour service and for house calls at night and on holidays as well as in the day time.

The services are rendered by a smaller or larger number of physicians and other members of the health professions who work together in systematic association, pooling their experience and skill, facilities and equipment, technical and other auxiliary personnel, operating expenses, and earnings. The persons covered by the plans are free to select their personal physician from among those on the staff of the group and to choose the group from which they wish to be attended if several units are affiliated with the plan. Establishment and maintenance of a personal relationship between the subscribers and their family physicians on the staff is given due attention.

The size and composition of the professional staffs vary greatly, depending upon the number of people regularly served, the special needs to be met, the type of community, and the internal organization of the unit. On the one extreme are large staffs consisting almost entirely of full-time personnel and including physicians, dentists, pharmacists, nurses, dieticians, laboratory technicians, X-ray technicians, physical therapists, medical social workers, health educators, optometrists, record librarians, and related professional persons in a varying number and combination. On the other extreme are plans which have only a small number of full-time physicians, nurses, and technicians and rely heavily on the systematic cooperation of part-time physicians representing various medical specialties and of part-time dentists and members of other health professions. In between is a multitude of arrangements which defy description.

The 56 groups surveyed by the United States Public Health Service in 1946 had a total of 622 full-time physicians, 258 part-time physicians, and 106 dentists. Only 31 of the groups had any part-time physicians and only 19 had dentists on their staffs. The medical staffs ranged in size from 3 to 95 physicians.[8]

Examples of plans with full-time or predominantly full-time medical staffs are the Northern Pacific Beneficial Association, Northern Pacific Railway Company, St. Paul, Minnesota and the Stanocola Employees' Medical and Hospital Association, Baton Rouge, Louisiana, both employee-administered industrial plans; the Tennessee Coal, Iron, and Railroad Company, Fairfield, Alabama, a company-administered industrial plan;

the Farmers' Union Hospital Association, Elk City, Oklahoma, and the Cooperative Hospital Association, Amherst, Texas, both rural consumer cooperatives; and the Milwaukee Medical Center, Milwaukee, Wisconsin, and the Ross-Loos Medical Group, Los Angeles, California, both private group clinics.

The policy of appointing a relatively larger number of part-time physicians in addition to a full-time staff is followed, among others, by the Consolidated Edison Employees' Mutual Aid Society, New York City, and the Gates Mutual Benefit Club, Denver, Colorado, both employee-administered plans in industry; and the Group Health Association, Washington, D.C., and the Labor Health Institute, St. Louis, Missouri, both organizations owned and controlled by the members.

The ratio of physicians to population is hard to determine, as a number of prepayment organizations make use of part-time physicians and render service to non-members who pay on the fee-for-service basis, to persons covered by Workmen's Compensation laws, or to both. Judging from the experience of some plans which serve mainly members of a prepayment plan and exclude care of legally compensable diseases and injuries, a group practice unit needs one full-time physician for about every thousand eligible persons. This ratio is subject to variations, depending not only upon the scope of the service offered but on the need and effective demand for medical care, preventive and curative.

In many units general practitioners and partial specialists constitute the majority of the staffs, in some the specialists are predominant, and in still others full specialists and general practitioners are represented about equally. The larger the number of people enrolled and the larger the size of the staff, the greater the number and variety of specialists that are serving full-time. This is illustrated by a comparison of the specialties represented on the staffs of the Stanocola Employees' Medical and Hospital Association, Baton Rouge, Louisiana, and the Ross-Loos Medical Group, Los Angeles, California, early in 1947. The first had 12 full-time physicians and several part-time physicians for approximately 19,000 participants, and the latter had 104 physicians to serve 99,840 participants and an unknown number of nonsubscribers.

Specialties Represented on the Staff of Two Group Practice Units

STANOCOLA ASSOCIATION	ROSS-LOOS MEDICAL GROUP
Obstetrics and gynecology	Allergy
Ophthalmology and otolaryngology	Dermatology
Pediatrics	Endocrinology
Radiology	Internal medicine, including cardiology, chest diseases, and gastroenterology
Surgery	Obstetrics
	Ophthalmology and otolaryngology
	Orthopedics
	Pediatrics
	Proctology
	Radiology
	Surgery, including general and special
	Urology

Whatever their practices in organizing the professional staffs, all plans bring general practitioners and specialists into the closest possible relations with each other and place emphasis on the utmost utilization of auxiliary personnel. Recently a tendency has appeared to vest responsibility for the patient in general practitioners or internists. They make the initial examination of new patients, refer them to the appropriate specialists, summarize all findings, make the final report, and take charge of the follow-up.

The Health Insurance Plan of Greater New York through a special committee of physicians has formulated minimum standards for the size of the medical groups, the composition of the staffs, the qualification of physicians representing the twelve specialties that are required, the physical facilities, and the organization of both services and administration.

The methods of paying the staff members are diverse. They depend on the type of appointments, the internal organization of the staff, and the policy in accepting patients other than those enrolled in the prepayment plan.

Regular staff members, part-time as well as full-time, usually receive fixed annual salaries graduated according to type of work, experience, and length of service. Additional income is not uncommon. The partners or shareholders of organizations controlled by physicians in private practice divide the profit either among themselves or among all regular staff members on the basis of widely varying schedules. Physicians affiliated with nonprofit organizations which also accept patients paying fees retain part of the income from this source or share in its distribution among all the doctors. The group practice units cooperating with the Health Insurance Plan of Greater New York receive from the plan a flat rate ("capitation fee") for each insured person enrolled with them and are free to distribute this money among the members of the unit as they choose.

In general the incomes of the individual physicians are net incomes, as their professional expenses are included in the common budget. Additional advantages usually offered by the plans are continuation of pay during sickness, vacation period, and leave of absence for postgraduate work; travel expenses to attend scientific meetings; and provision for liability, life, and accident insurance. Retirement benefits have been introduced recently by some organizations.

Organization of hospital care.—Hospitalization is either furnished in organization-owned facilities or made readily available in those community hospitals with which the individual physicians on the staff of the group are affiliated or the group as such has made an agreement. Plans not covering hospital care recently have tended to utilize the services of Blue Cross organizations on the basis of more or less formal understandings and in such cases expect their members to join the Blue Cross plan as well.

Some nonprofit plans, chiefly those in rural areas, have raised the capital funds for the construction and equipment of hospitals of their own by requesting prospective members to buy shares of stock or pay a—transferable—life membership fee ranging from $25 to $50. This idea has fallen on fruitful soil in varying parts of the country, after it had proved its feasibility and value in Elk City, Oklahoma. There the farmers, remembering their favorable experience with a cooperative cotton gin, gladly accepted the suggestion to apply the cooperative principle to the building of a hospital.[9]

Prepayment rates.—The prepayments cover either most of the services or selected services only. They apply to the care of family dependents as well as breadwinners or to that of subscribers only.

The rates are set according to the scope of the services offered, graduated according to the size of the family, and are usually somewhat higher for persons not enrolling in groups. The prevailing policy is to charge flat rates rather than percentages of the income of the subscribers, one of the exceptions being the Labor Health Institute, St. Louis, Missouri. In most instances the prepayments of group subscribers are due monthly and those of individual subscribers at least quarterly. The rural plans often require annual, semiannual, or quarterly payments in advance.

If the prepayment rates do not cover all the available services, extra charges are made for specified types of care, service to family dependents, or both. Additional charges of relatively small amounts are common for home calls and night calls. In some instances application fees, initial membership fees, or both are required.

The costs are borne by the subscribers alone in the majority of all cases and by employers and employees jointly in the minority. The employers pay the full contributions for their employees in the case of the Labor Health Institute, St. Louis, Missouri, and one half in the case of the Health Insurance Plan of Greater New York, the city government matching the payments of municipal employees.

In 1946, the prepayment rates charged by the various plans ranged from $16 to $48 a year for one person and from $34 to $96 a year for the whole family, depending on the scope of service and type of enrollment. Individual subscribers paid from 10 to 20 per cent more than group subscribers.

Administration.—According to the structure of their administrative organization, the group practice prepayment plans may be classified in four categories: physician-controlled, company-administered, consumer cooperatives, and associations directed by representatives of all groups in the community. The first two place all administrative responsibility in representatives of the owners of the institutions, on the theory that the subscribers are merely signatories to a contract. The last two give subscribers seat and voice in the administrative bodies. They grant those who are eligible for service and those who are to render it the right to participate in management, each group in its own field. All plans vest medical directors with full authority for the professional services, including the appointment of professional personnel, and employ business managers or executive secretaries and a varying number of clerical personnel.

The cooperatives and the plans which are cooperative in structure are administered by boards of trustees (or directors) and officers who are elected by the members from the members and serve without remuneration. Annual membership meetings and regular meetings of the directors and officers are the rule. Nearly all organizations employ paid executives.

The widely used term "consumer-control" must not be construed as meaning lay control of professional matters. The professional independence of the physicians and dentists and the protection of the patient-doctor relationship are assured by specific provisions in the bylaws of most of the associations. These state explicitly that neither the board of directors nor the membership shall supervise, regulate, or intervene in the professional relationship between the physicians and their patients. An illustration of this policy is afforded by the bylaws of the Group Health Association, Washington, D.C., which declare:

The Board of Trustees shall in no way regulate or supervise the practice of medicine by any physician with whom it contracts for the care of members, nor shall it in any way supervise, regulate, or interfere with the usual professional relationship between such physician and his patient-member, and every such contract entered into by and between a physician and the Association shall contain a positive covenant to that effect.

EXAMPLES OF INDUSTRIAL PLANS

The prepayment plan of the *Tennessee Coal, Iron, and Railroad Company* in Fairfield, Alabama, was established in 1913 by the company. It is part and parcel of a comprehensive system of health and welfare activities at the plant, including safety and sanitation programs, health education, medical care, financial assistance through a credit union, disability insurance through a mutual benefit association, and provisions for retirement and life insurance. The facilities and services for medical care are designed for the care of patients with injuries and diseases compensable under the Workmen's Compensation law as well as for service to persons covered by the prepayment plan.

The company employees with incomes of less than $3,000, their family dependents, and pensioners of the company are eligible to join the organization. There are no age restrictions. Medical examination is not required.

The prepayment plan provides for the services of physicians at the home (restricted to those living within the area and subscribing to the "district service"), at the clinic, and at the hospital, including all specialist services, periodic health examinations of children and adults, vaccinations, immunizations, and maternity services; mouth examinations for both adults and children and dental treatment for school children referred after annual examination; clinical laboratory services; diagnostic roentgenological services for school children taking the annual health examination; ordinary drugs, anesthetics, and dressings; and home nursing. Additional services are available at extra charge. They include dental treatment of adults, diagnostic X-ray examinations of others than school children, therapeutic roentgenological services, physiotherapy, drugs other than ordinary, medical and surgical appliances, hospitalization in wards (at low rates), use of the operating and delivery rooms, clinical laboratory and X-ray services in the hospital, and ambulance service. Eyeglasses are obtainable at discount.

The company has built and maintains a general hospital with 273 beds and 42 bassinets and a large out-patient department and 13 "dispensaries" in eight districts around the works and the villages. The hospital is equipped for all specialist services and used as a clearing house and center of all the work of the company's health department. It is approved by the American College of Surgeons as meeting its requirements and approved by the Council on Hospitals and Medical Education of the American Medical Association for residencies as well as for intern training. The dispensaries serve as first-aid stations and centers of the district service, providing general medical care for all ambulatory patients, home care for subscribers, and preventive health services for infants. The typical dispensary has two treatment rooms, two rooms for dental service, two office rooms, one waiting room, and one bedroom for the physician on call.

A large staff of full-time professional and related personnel is employed by the company. The medical staff is utilized for pre-employment examinations, plant supervision, preventive health services, first-aid service, care of patients with compensable injuries and diseases, and service to members of the prepayment plan. The specialists assigned to the base hospital and the out-patient department act as consultants to the general practitioners stationed at the dispensaries. There is no recent information on the total number of professional and related personnel.

The company supports the services in the plant and the villages and the care of patients with compensable injuries and diseases. It contributes to the cost of the prepayment plan. The present rates and extra charges cannot be stated, due to lack of information.

The administration of the prepayment plan as well as of all other health services is in the hands of the company, which maintains a health department with four subdivisions: the sanitary, medical, dental, and base hospital divisions. This agency is under the direction of a Chief Surgeon and Superintendent, who is responsible directly and solely to the president of the corporation and has complete control over the management of all services.

The *Stanocola Employees' Medical and Hospital Association* at Baton Rouge, Louisiana, was organized in 1924 by employees of the Standard Oil Company at its refinery at Baton Rouge. The organization was incorporated in 1930 under the nontrading laws of Louisiana.

The association accepts employees of the company after one year of continuous service. Membership covers wives and dependent children, including stepchildren and adopted children. Dependent male children are eligible for the services until they reach the age of twenty-one and beyond this age while going to school. Female children are entitled to the services regardless of age, so long as they meet the dependency requirement. Dependent parents, including stepparents, and any other relatives of the member or of his wife are also entitled to service, provided they meet the dependency requirement. In the case of relatives other than parents a slight addition to the regular monthly prepayments is required. All relatives must wait three months before being entitled to service, with the exception of parents, whose waiting period is six months. No income restrictions are placed on enrollment. Medical examination is not required for membership.

The number of members has risen from 2,200 in April, 1924, to 5,200, representing about 19,700 persons, in April, 1947. About 80 per cent of all eligible employees are enrolled.

The prepayment plan covers the services of general practitioners and specialists at the home, clinic, and hospital, including vaccinations and immunizations, maternity services, and preventive services for children; routine clinical laboratory tests; diagnostic roentgenological services, including dental examinations; physiotherapy; electrocardiograms; dressings and certain medical and surgical appliances; and hospitalization and private duty nursing in the hospital and home up to a total cost of $250 per case of sickness. Home calls are made within a radius of seven miles of the city limits. Drugs may be purchased at considerable advantage through special arrangements with a pharmacy operating a drug counter in the clinic building.

The association owns, debt free, a two-story clinic building centrally located in the city of Baton Rouge and utilizes the two nonprofit hospitals in the community. The medical staff consists of sixteen physicians, including three surgeons, two eye, ear, nose, and throat specialists, one obstetrician and gynecologist, one internist, one pediatrician, one general practitioner with special attention to radiology, and seven general practitioners. In addition, there are three graduate nurses, four nongraduate nurses, two laboratory technicians, two X-ray technicians, one physiotherapist, four receptionists and office workers, and janitorial help. House calls at present are being made by physicians in the community, who are compensated on a fee basis. Recently limited physicians' service has been tried out in two congested outlying rural communities, and this service has now been instituted successfully in one of these areas.

The monthly prepayment rate is $5.00, covering the member and his eligible dependents in the classes of wives, children, and parents. An additional payment of $1.00 per month is made for covered dependents outside of these three classes. Every new member must pay an initiation fee of $20.00 in monthly installments of $1.00. Originally the association had issued a capital stock of 5,000 shares of a value of $20.00 each and required every member to buy and hold one share. The company has always accorded the organization the privilege of payroll deduction and, since the inauguration of an employees' thrift plan, has granted it the right of dues payment through employee-members' savings accounts, which are jointly maintained in this plan by the company and the employees.

The affairs of the association are managed by a board of eleven directors, elected for two-year overlapping terms by popular vote of the employee-members and serving without remuneration. Eight of the directors are elected by members in various departments of the plant and three from the group at large. The officers are elected annually by the board, the secretary being the only paid member of the administrative body. Responsibility for all professional matters is vested in the medical director. Appointment of medical personnel is made by the board with the advice and recommendation of the medical director.

The *Gates Mutual Benefit Club*, Denver, Colorado, a non-profit organization, was founded in 1929 by the employees of the Gates Rubber Company "for the purpose of extending mutual assistance and the establishment of friendly interests among the employees . . . and of furthering any other activities for the advancement of the economic, financial and social welfare of members and employees." Its functions are confined to benefits and services for conditions not covered by the Workmen's Compensation law.

All employees are eligible, regardless of age and income. Inclusion of family dependents is under consideration. All new employees of the company who apply for membership must pass a "complete physical examination," the passing of the usual pre-employment examination being regarded as sufficient. The executive committee of the organization has the right to reject any application if this is deemed "advisable for the good of the Club" but rarely makes use of the authorization. Employees who retire from the company upon reaching the age of retirement and have been members of the club for at least five years immediately preceding retirement are eligible for specified medical and related services. Medical care is furnished under the plan after thirty days of membership. Tonsillectomies and the discount allowed on eye refraction and purchase of eyeglasses are available after six-months. No service is rendered for maternity, chronic conditions existing at the time of employment, venereal diseases, disorders due to alcoholism, any type of illness resulting from complications of pregnancy, and "pelvic cases" among female employees during the first year of membership and hospitalization of such cases regardless of the period of membership.

Early in 1947 approximately 5,800 of the 6,000 company employees in Denver were club members.

The benefits include weekly disability benefits after the seventh calendar day of illness, a funeral benefit, and medical, dental, hospital, and related services.

The medical care program makes provision for the services of staff physicians—specialists as well as general practitioners—at the home, clinic, and hospital; all necessary diagnostic laboratory tests, X-ray services, and electrocardiography; eye examinations and fitting of glasses, with the club paying part of the costs of refraction and glasses; prescribed medicines and drugs; allowances of up to $10 toward the cost of prescribed belts, braces, or supports; mouth examinations by dentists, dental X-ray examinations when considered necessary by the dentist, cleaning, extractions, emergency treatments, pyorrhea treatment, treatment of trench mouth and other forms of gum diseases, and temporary (cement) fillings; hospitalization in a semiprivate room up to ten weeks in any twelve-month period, including general nursing, clinical laboratory and roentgenological services, use of the operating room, anesthesia, dressings, splints, special drugs, and blood transfusions; and ambulance service when ordered by a staff physician.

The plan operates from a company-owned clinic building, staffed with full-time and part-time personnel. Bed-patients are taken to a local hospital. In addition, there is a first-aid station located inside the plant. Early in 1947 the staff consisted of five full-time general practitioners, five part-time specialists, three full-time dentists, one full-time pharmacist, ten registered nurses, one full-time and one part-time laboratory technician, and six clerks, receptionists, and office workers.

The weekly prepayment rate in 1947 was $0.45, of which $0.35 was for medical care and $0.10 for sickness benefits. The dues are deducted from the pay checks. The company contributes to the operation of the plan by providing the building, including its maintenance and repair, the utilities, and some money for services rendered. The budget for 1947 was in excess of $150,000.

Administrative responsibility is vested in a board of directors and an executive committee. Of the seventeen board members, fifteen are elected by popular vote of the club members and two are ex officio members, the treasurer and the assistant treasurer, who are appointed by the company. The executive committee consists of elected officers of the club and is charged with the duty of passing on all applications for membership, awarding sick and funeral benefits, and transacting other routine business. The general administration of all club activities is in the hands of a manager, who also represents the company. He and the personnel director of the corporation sit in on all meetings of the board of directors and important meetings of the executive committee. A medical director has full authority for the assignment of all professional personnel and for the services rendered under the plan, including the final decision on the interpretation of the bylaws in regard to medical care.

EXAMPLES OF COOPERATIVES OUTSIDE INDUSTRY

The *Farmers' Union Hospital Association* at Elk City, Oklahoma, was organized in 1929 through the joint efforts of Dr. Michael A. Shadid and a group of farmers. In the same year it was incorporated as a nonprofit association under the Cooperative and Benevolent Laws of Oklahoma.

Membership in the organization is open to any person whose application is approved by the board of directors. Neither age restrictions nor income limitations are applied. Medical examination is required. Family dependents as well as subscribers are eligible. The term family dependent is interpreted as meaning "father, mother, and all unmarried children living at home and relying on the family for food, clothing and shelter." Other relatives may be included in place of one member of the family if it consists of less than four persons. Patients not covered by the plan may obtain service at regular fees. The money received for their care goes into the hospital fund. In April, 1947, the organization had 2,800 subscribers representing approximately 9,500 persons. Many nonsubscribers utilize the services of the association.

The plan provides for specified services without additional charges and for others at low rates. In the first category are all diagnostic and treatment services, including prenatal, obstetrical, and postnatal care, for ambulatory and hospitalized patients by staff physicians; routine laboratory tests; fluoroscopic X-ray examinations; and ultraviolet, infrared, diathermy, radium, and X-ray treatment. Hospital care in semiprivate accommodations of the Community Hospital of the organization is available at the daily rate of $5.00 for first-year members and of $3.00 for members enrolled for more than one full year. The charges for anesthetics and the use of the operating room range from $10 to $20. Dental care is offered at prices ranging from $0.50 for an X-ray picture of the teeth or an extraction to $55 for dentures (lucitone). The professional fee for a home call is $1.00 and the charge for mileage 20 cents per mile each way, plus $1.00 for night calls.

The association owns a three-storied 100-bed hospital, which has evolved out of the original red brick building with twenty beds, a nurses' home, and a heating and laundry plant. It is planning to add a clinic building. The cost of construction and equipment have been defrayed by the sale of member shares in the amount of $50 and the fees paid by nonsubscribers.

The personnel in 1947 numbered sixty-four, including six physicians, one dentist, one pharmacist, eight registered nurses, twenty-two practical nurses, three laboratory and X-ray technicians, and twenty-three others. The medical staff consisted of six full-time physicians, including two general practitioners and four specialists representing gynecology and obstetrics, ophthalmology and otorhinolaryngology, surgery and orthopedics, and urology. The salaries of the staff physicians ranged from $4,200 to $8,400 a year and were supplemented by the payment of a bonus.

The annual prepayment rates charged in 1947 were $16 for one person, $24 for a couple, $30 for three persons, and $34 for a family of four or more.

The organization is administered by a board of five directors, charged with the duty of exercising, conducting, and controlling "the corporate powers, business and property of the Association," and elected officers, all serving without remuneration. The directors are elected by the members at the annual meeting. All must be members of the association. No person on the staff of the hospital or clinic or other employee can qualify as a director during the time of his connection with the plan. The medical director has full authority for the direction and supervision of the professional services.

The *Group Health Association*, Washington, D.C., was organized in 1937 as a nonprofit corporation under the law governing the organization of charitable, educational, and religious associations in the District of Columbia.

Eligibility is extended to individuals as well as groups of employed persons regardless of income and age. Groups consist of a suitable percentage of persons employed by a single employer, in one administrative unit of a business firm or governmental agency, or in one building or office. The percentage of those who must join to obtain service under the group agreement varies according to the size of the basic unit, ranging from 100 per cent for units of five to six persons to 50 per cent for units with more than fifty persons. Members of a group meeting the requirements are accepted without medical examination. Individual applicants must pass a medical examination and pay an application fee of $2.00 for themselves, plus $2.00 for each dependent listed on their application. Family dependents as well as breadwinners are eligible. Family dependents are the wife or husband, the children up to eighteen years of age, and any persons receiving their major support from the member.

The prepayment plan covers all services specified in the agreement except care of conditions furnished under specific laws. Upon request, the staff is ready to treat members entitled to care under the Workmen's Compensation law or the provisions for veterans. Maternity service is subject to a waiting period of ten months but is furnished at nominal cost before that time. Elective surgery is available under the same conditions.

Excluded are brain and nerve surgery, plastic surgery, correction of deformities and birthmarks, psychiatric treatment, chiropody, deep or intermediate X-ray and radium therapy, and treatment of tuberculosis, mental disease, drug addiction, and alcoholism after the need for hospital care has been determined by the medical director. Dental care is not available at present but is under consideration for introduction at the earliest possible date.

The total number of participants has risen from 4,874 at the end of 1938 to 12,216 in March, 1947.

The organization offers two types of plans, one providing for full service as specified in the agreement and the other one covering medical attention but not hospitalization.

Persons eligible for full service are entitled to the services of staff physicians—specialists as well as general practitioners—including preventive services, health examinations, and prenatal, obstetrical, and postnatal care, at the home, clinic, and hospital; all clinical laboratory tests; diagnostic and therapeutic X-ray services; physiotherapy; eye examinations and prescriptions; and hospitalization (semiprivate service) up to sixty days in any calendar year or any one illness or condition. Hospital care includes general nursing, routine laboratory examinations, use of the operating or delivery room, anesthesia, dressings and most medications, nursery care, emergency room facilities, and the use of an ambulance if requested by the attending physician. The first $50 of the costs of hospital service for maternity must be paid by the member. For the first home call in any illness $1.00 is charged if the call is within an airline radius of eight miles from the clinic and $2.00 if it is within a radius of eight to fifteen miles. Subsequent home calls in the same case of illness are made without charge. The cost of drugs and materials used in caring for ambulatory patients are to be paid by the members.

Members who have taken the limited plan must have made

Group Practice Plans

arrangements for hospitalization through another nonprofit prepayment plan or a commercial insurance company.

Individual subscribers may not receive plan service for conditions present at the time of admission but in such cases can obtain care, except for hospitalization, upon payment of nominal fees.

All members are offered the opportunity to buy prescribed medicines, drugs, and supplies at the pharmacies of the association and to obtain eyeglasses and frames at reduced cost.

The association operates clinics at two locations in the District of Columbia and utilizes all the hospitals in the community that are available to the public.

The total number of full-time personnel on July 1, 1947, was eighty-one, including thirteen physicians, three registered pharmacists, fifteen registered nurses, three practical nurses, seven laboratory, X-ray, physical therapy, and optical technicians, and forty other persons (including one optometrist). In addition to the full-time medical staff, eleven physicians were serving on a part-time basis. Seven physicians were engaged in general practice and internal medicine, and seventeen represented the following specialties: allergy (one), dermatology (one), neurology (one), obstetrics and gynecology (three), ophthalmology (one), otolaryngology (one), pediatrics (four), roentgenology (one), and surgery (four).

The monthly prepayments for subscribers to the full service in 1947 were $3.00 for the subscriber, $3.00 for the adult dependent, and $2.00 for each of the first three dependent children, with additional children accepted without charge. The corresponding figures for the service without hospitalization were $2.50, $2.50, and $1.75, respectively. A discount of 5 per cent is given to group members if a single payment is made for the whole group and to individual members if they pay on an annual basis. Each member must share in the cost of equipment by contributing a "membership fee" of $10.00, which may be paid in monthly rates of $1.00, together with the regular dues.

The association is administered by a board of nine trustees, elected from the membership by the membership, and elected officers, all serving without remuneration. An advisory council assists the board, and paid personnel, including one executive director, is employed for the management. The medical director of the organization has full responsibility for all professional matters, including the appointment of physicians and the supervision of the services.

In 1946, more than four fifths of the income of the association was derived from dues and nearly one tenth from the operation of the pharmacy. Salaries and fees of physicians accounted for more than one third of the expenses, other clinic salaries for about one fifth, hospitalization for nearly one sixth, and office and administrative salaries for more than one seventh.

EXAMPLES OF PHYSICIAN-CONTROLLED PLANS

The *Ross-Loos Medical Group* in Los Angeles, California, was organized in 1929 by Drs. Donald E. Ross and H. Clifford Loos. It started with a contract to serve employees of the Los Angeles City Department of Water and Power and their families, soon obtained additional subscribers from other departments of the municipal government, industrial corporations, and mercantile firms, and grew to become the largest group practice prepayment plan under the auspices of physicians in private practice.

The plan accepts employed persons enrolling in groups regardless of age and also permits individual enrollment of "any person of the Caucasian race" between the ages of twenty-one and fifty, inclusive. There is no income limit for eligibility. Persons enrolling in groups may be accepted without medical examination, although the right to request such an examination is reserved by the Group. Acceptance of subscribers under the system of individual enrollment is dependent on "satisfactory physical examination given by a staff member" of the Group. The subscribers must be located within a radius of fifteen miles of one of the designated offices of the Group.

The "agreement" to be signed by group subscribers and the organization states that

the Subscribing Group hereby engages the services of the Medical Group [a copartnership of physicians and surgeons duly licensed to practice medicine and surgery in the State of California] to render medical and surgical care and attention to the members of the Subscribing Group who subscribe for said service in accordance with the covenants and conditions hereinafter provided for the sum of . . . per month for each subscriber of the Subscribing Group. Payment shall be made by the Subscribing Group, as agent for all its subscriber members, on the . . . day of each month for the preceding month.

The services of the Group are also available to the family dependents of the subscribers at specified low rates set forth in a schedule and to nonsubscribers on the fee-for-service basis at rates approximating those prevailing in the area.

The total number of subscribers was nearly 6,000 by the end of 1930, more than 12,000 by the end of 1935, about 26,000 by the end of 1940, and 31,200 by the end of 1946. Persons covered by group contracts constituted about four fifths of the enrollment, and many were municipal employees. The family dependents of subscribers numbered 68,640 as of December 31, 1946.

Unless eligible for treatment under the California Workmen's Compensation law, the persons covered by the prepayment plan are entitled to the full services of physicians—specialists as well as general practitioners—at the home, clinic, and hospital, including routine health examinations, prenatal and postnatal care, and consultations; eye refractions; all clinical laboratory services; X-ray examinations exclusive of dental examinations; physiotherapy; all prescribed medicines, drugs, and dressings; anesthesia; hospitalization in a hospital designated by the Group up to ninety days in any period of twelve consecutive months, including accommodation in a two-bed room or, if ordered by the physician, a private room, general nursing, meals and special diets, all clinical laboratory and diagnostic X-ray services, electrocardiograms, operating room, anesthetics, surgical supplies, dressings, splints and casts, drugs, oxygen, and physiotherapy; and ambulance service for a distance not to exceed fifteen miles traveled by a patient on any one trip. X-ray therapy services are furnished at nominal rates. Excluded are treatment of subscribers with self-inflicted illness or injuries, drug addiction, and alcoholism; medication and prophylaxis for patients with venereal disease; dental care; radium treatment; eyeglasses; hospitalization for cases of obstetrics, abortions, miscarriages, venereal disease, mental disease, alcoholism, drug addiction or conditions arising therefrom; and rest-home cures.

The Group owns a thirteen-story building in downtown Los Angeles and nine centers in various sections of the metropolitan area. In addition, it rents three centers and utilizes two "associated offices." The main building serves as headquarters and houses most of the specialist divisions, while the other centers are equipped to perform the services ordinarily rendered by general practitioners and internists.

The staff has grown from three physicians, including the two founders and one salaried general practitioner, in 1929 to an organization with a total of 338 persons at the end of 1946. These included 98 full-time physicians, 6 registered pharmacists, 118 registered nurses, 5 optometrists, 4 X-ray technicians, 6 physiotherapists, 2 anesthetists, and other personnel. Of the 98 physicians, 43 were general practitioners and 55 represented 13 specialties: internal medicine (14), surgery (9), obstetrics and gynecology (6), otorhinolaryngology (6), ophthalmology (5), pediatrics (4), dermatology (3), urology (3), and allergy, endocrinology, neurology, pathology, and roentgenology (1

Group Practice Plans

each). By April, 1947, the medical staff consisted of 104 full-time physicians, the additions including one general practitioner, one internist, one orthopedic surgeon, one proctologist, one pediatrician, and one surgeon.

The Group has access to most of the local hospitals but for reasons of convenience uses mainly the Queen of Angels Hospital, a nonprofit general hospital with 525 beds which is approved by the American College of Surgeons as meeting unconditionally its minimum standards, approved for training interns by the Council on Medical Education and Hospitals of the American Medical Association, and accredited as a school of nursing by the State Board of Nurse Examiners.

All staff physicians are permitted to attend nonsubscribers desiring their services and to charge them at their discretion. Of the collections from service to nonsubscribers, one half is credited to the attending physicians and the other half turned over to the organization. The income of the physicians is derived from the basic salary, the bonus distributed annually, and the fees paid by nonsubscribers. The profits of the organization are divided among the sixteen partners, the two founders receiving approximately 15 per cent each and the other fourteen approximately 5 per cent each. The partnership agreement provides for the acquisition of the holdings of retiring or deceased partners by other members.

The monthly prepayment rate for group subscribers is $3.00 and that for individual subscribers $4.00. The latter also pay an examination fee of $2.00 and a registration fee of $4.00.

Examples of "dependent fees" are $50.00 for a maternity case, including prenatal and postnatal care, $25.00 for major surgery, $15.00 for minor surgery, $5.00 for an electrocardiogram, $2.00 for a gastric analysis, $1.50 for a home call (day), and $0.75 for a clinic call, ordinary laboratory tests, or a physiotherapy treatment. The family dependents are responsible for their own hospital bills.

Administrative control is exercised by a partnership committee, which is assisted by several other committees, including the scientific, finance, personnel, purchasing, housing, and maintenance committees. The organization employs a business manager, who sits in on meetings of the committees, and clerical personnel numbering about eighty in 1947.

The *Trinity Hospital,* Little Rock, Arkansas, as early as 1924 had group prepayment contracts in force with several business organizations but later had to terminate them. The present prepayment plan dates back to 1931.

Membership is open to employed persons enrolling in groups and their family dependents and also to persons subscribing as individuals. There are neither age nor income restrictions. No physical examination is required. In addition to subscribers, other persons are accepted for service at the regular fees.

The organization had 2,544 contracts covering 6,101 persons in 1940 and 2,153 contracts covering 5,016 persons early in 1947. The decline, caused by the loss of physicians during the war, has been halted and expansion has begun lately.

Eligibility for service does not extend to "the care or treatment of purposely self-inflicted injury, eye, mental, alcoholic, dental, or rest-cure cases" nor of pre-existing diseases or conditions during the first year of membership except for acute conditions needing immediate attention. Elective surgery is subject to a waiting period of twelve months. Hospitalization is not furnished for patients with diseases for which the hospital is not equipped to care and which it does not under ordinary circumstances accept, including pulmonary tuberculosis, marked mental or nervous disorders, drug addictions, or diseases quarantinable by the city, county, or state authorities. However, preliminary hospitalization for diagnostic purposes is provided when deemed advisable in the opinion of a staff member. Maternity care is available after ten months of membership.

The "agreements for annual hospitalization, surgical and

medical service" are of two types. The first provides the subscribers and their family dependents with all the services of physicians—specialists as well as general practitioners—at the headquarters of the organization, including consultations, smallpox vaccinations, immunizations against typhoid and diphtheria, and maternity care; all routine laboratory tests; roentgenological examinations and treatments; radium treatment; and hospitalization in a two-bed room of the Trinity Hospital up to six weeks in any one year, including general nursing, meals and diets, routine laboratory work, use of the operating room, anesthesia, dressings, splints, and all ordinary medicines and drugs prescribed. The agreement does not cover home calls; orthopedic appliances; insulin, sera, vaccines, drugs or appliances deemed expensive beyond the spirit of the agreement; and special nursing in the hospital. Home calls are made at the charge of $2.00 for a day call and $4.00 for a night call (between 8 p.m. and 7 a.m.).

The second type of agreement covers the regular services for subscribers but only hospital care for family dependents, with reduced fees for specified professional services including surgery, laboratory tests, roentgenological examinations, physiotherapy, and deep X-ray therapy.

The comprehensive contract is taken by the large majority of all subscribers. Early in 1947, approximately nine out of ten plan members were enrolled under the "full coverage" contract.

The organization owns and operates a fifty-bed hospital with an out-patient department. All physicians are on full-time salary. In April, 1947, the total full-time personnel numbered seventy, including eight physicians, one pharmacist, fourteen registered nurses, two laboratory and X-ray technicians, and forty-five other personnel. The medical specialties represented included internal medicine (2), obstetrics (2), pediatrics (2), surgery (2), and urology and otolaryngology (1 each).

The monthly prepayment rates for group subscribers to the contract covering full service for family dependents as well as subscribers in 1947 were $2.00 for the subscriber, $2.50 for the spouse, $2.00 for the first child, $1.50 for the second child, and a maximum of $8.00 for a family of four or more. The monthly rates for group subscribers to the contract covering full service for the subscriber and limited service for his family dependents were $2.00 for the subscriber, $1.25 for the spouse, $0.75 for the first child, $0.50 for the second child, and a maximum of $4.50 for a family of four or more.

The "non-group rates" were fifty cents higher on any of the types of contract and payable quarterly, semi-annually, or annually, with 5 per cent and 10 per cent discount being given for semi-annual and annual payments, respectively.

Typical charges for family dependents are $25.00 for major surgery or obstetrical services; $10.00 for minor surgery; $2.00 for a home call, blood chemistry, basal metabolism, or electrocardiogram; $1.00 for a malaria test or a physiotherapy treatment; and $0.50 for an office call or an ordinary laboratory test.

The administration is in the hands of the seven partners, who employ a business manager and nine clerical personnel.

THE HEALTH INSURANCE PLAN OF GREATER NEW YORK

The Health Insurance Plan of Greater New York (HIP) was incorporated in 1944 under Article IX–C of the Insurance Law of the State of New York and began operation early in 1947.

It accepts all persons employed in New York City earning a base wage or salary of not more than $5,000 a year and their dependents, regardless of age and without prior medical examination. Dependents are defined by state law as spouse and unmarried children under eighteen years of age. At least 75 per cent of the eligible employees in a firm or a division must sign up to make enrollment effective, and there must be a minimum of twenty-five insured employees in an enrollment group.

In addition, the present underwriting rules of HIP state that the employer must agree to contribute at least half of the total cost of the insurance for his employees and their family dependents. Persons enrolled with HIP must also carry adequate hospitalization insurance (Associated Hospital Service of New York City or the substantial equivalent).

The HIP program provides for general medical, specialist, surgical, and obstetrical care at the home, office, and hospital; diagnostic and laboratory procedures; periodic health examinations, immunizations, and other preventive measures; physical therapy, radiotherapy, and other therapeutic services; professional services for the administration of blood plasma; eye examinations; visiting nurse service at the home; ambulance service from the home to the hospital; and psychiatric examination and consultation. It excludes medical service for acute alcoholism, drug addiction, ailments requiring long-term or institutional treatment, treatment by a psychiatrist, purely cosmetic surgery, dental care, prescribed drugs, appliances, and eyeglasses.

The professional services are rendered by group practice units composed of licensed physicians who have entered into an agreement with HIP. Stimulation of an active interest among physicians to band together and form groups has been one of the foremost objectives of the plan. By the end of May, 1947, there were 22 medical groups participating, with a total of 545 physicians. Each medical group contains, in addition to general physicians, qualified specialists in at least the following twelve fields: internal medicine, general surgery, obstetrics-gynecology, pediatrics, otolaryngology, ophthalmology, urology, orthopedics, dermatology, neuropsychiatry, roentgenology, and pathology. Physicians are not required to limit their practice to HIP subscribers.

A "Medical Control Board" of the organization examines each group's application for a contract. The control board is composed of fifteen physicians representing organized medicine, participating medical groups, and the board of directors of HIP. Each medical group that applies is examined for minimum professional qualifications and for business and legal aspects. Each insured person is free to choose among the participating medical groups serving his area of residence and to select his personal physician from among those who are members of the group chosen. The medical control board also has responsibility for the maintenance of satisfactory professional standards in the operation of the program.

HIP stresses a broad definition of health and illness, mental as well as physical. With the assistance of auxiliary medical and social service personnel, the medical groups are to give fullest attention to the social, economic, and emotional components of health and disease among all insured persons under their care. An intensive program of health education is in process of development.

The monthly prepayment rates in force in 1947 were $2.42 for single subscribers, $4.84 for a couple, and $7.25 for a family, regardless of the number of children. The prepayments are shared equally by employers and employees. The municipality of New York has assumed responsibility for payment of one half of the rates of both the Health Insurance Plan and the Associated Hospital Service for those of its employees and their dependents who wish to join. The United Nations has made a similar agreement for its staff. Several unions with health and welfare funds have also joined, and private industry is showing marked interest.

As of July 1, 1947, approximately 60,000 persons were enrolled, about equally divided between subscribers and family dependents.

Administrative responsibility is vested in a board of twenty-four directors representing medicine, labor, business, city government, and social welfare. The executive officers include a medical director and a general manager.

Group Practice Plans 181

EXPERIENCE AND APPRAISAL

Experience.—Most group practice prepayment plans have steadily increased in membership. In recent years many were unable to accept all the applicants because of the war-created difficulties in obtaining the necessary number of additional staff members and in expanding their physical facilities. This very fact indicates the growing reputation of the group practice units in many communities and the subscribers' satisfaction with both the service received and the personal relationship established with staff physicians and dentists.

Detailed data on the experience gained in operation of the organizations are few. Much valuable material has remained buried in files, and important sources of information have never been tapped. However, the findings of the few field studies that have been made, the observations of many professional persons, and the statistics published in annual reports permit certain broad conclusions.

The amount of services received by plan members differs markedly from organization to organization. In three prepayment plans the annual number of specified services per eligible person in the years 1938 and 1939, respectively, was as follows: attendance at the clinic, from 4 to 13; home visits, from 0.12 to 1.8; admissions to general hospitals, from 0.09 to 0.12; and days of hospitalization from 0.6 to 0.7.[10]

A detailed analysis of the services rendered during the period of July, 1940, to June, 1941, by a physician-owned organization in a southern city to persons enrolled in its prepayment plan yielded the following data. The annual number of services per eligible person was 5.5 for attendance at the clinic, 0.16 for home visits, and 0.08 for hospitalization. The monthly averages per 1,000 eligible persons were 459.6 clinic calls (including 352.7 physician calls and 106.9 calls for the services of nurses or laboratory technicians only), 367.2 visits to physicians (indicating that more than one physician was consulted during one clinic call), 13.2 home calls, and 73.3 days of hospitalization. Over the months the rate of clinic calls was relatively stable, but home calls and days of hospitalization varied considerably.[11]

The average length of hospital stay of the members of three prepayment plans ranged from 5 to 8 days in 1938 and 1939, respectively. In the Permanente Health Plans it was 7.7 days and 7.0 days in 1943 and 1944, respectively, as compared with 6.7 and 5.7 days, respectively, for patients paying directly, and 10.7 and 9.7 days, respectively, for patients treated under the Workmen's Compensation law.[12]

The Labor Health Institute in St. Louis reported an average stay of 8.2 days for subscribers and 8.6 days for family dependents in 1946, and the Group Health Association of Washington an average stay of 8.1 days per eligible person in 1946.

It is generally observed that plan members tend to call at the clinic to ask what they could do to keep well and to seek advice for minor ailments, and that patients with acute conditions come under care without delay. In a number of instances, more than one third of the clinic services consisted of specialists' services. Several plans report unusually low case fatality rates for such diseases as pneumonia, acute appendicitis, and perforated stomach ulcer.

The total average costs, including extra charges as well as prepayments and administrative as well as service expenses, ranged from about $11 to $30 per eligible person in three plans in 1938 and 1939, reflecting variations in scope of service, composition of membership, and age of the programs.[13] They were estimated at approximately $19 per person enrolled in a southern plan in 1940-1941 [14] and at about $30 per person covered by the Permanente Health Service in 1945.[15] Substantially all of the subscribers pay an amount close to the average. The administrative expenses, excluding nonoperating expenses, are reasonable, considering the broad scope of the

Group Practice Plans

services. In some instances they were below 10 per cent of the total costs and in others between 10 and 15 per cent.

The experience of well-established group practice prepayment plans of unquestionable adequacy permits estimates of the total average cost of such medical care programs at the price levels existing at the end of 1946. Medical care, including hospitalization in general hospitals as well as all medical and related services but excluding dental care and prescribed drugs, may cost from $25 to $30 per person and year. These figures are computed on the assumption that there is one full-time physician for every thousand eligible persons (lower figure) or one full-time physician for every nine hundred eligible persons (higher figure); that the average net income of the general practitioner is $8,000 and that of the specialists $14,000; that the average cost of the hospital day (general hospital) is $9.50; and that the treatment of patients with long-term conditions is limited in period.

The average net incomes of the physicians affiliated with prepayment plans ranged from about $3,000 for physicians in assistant positions to about $10,000 for specialists and medical directors in the late thirties and were considerably higher in the early forties. The physicians serving on the staff of the Farmers' Union Hospital Association, Elk City, Oklahoma, in 1946 had an average salary of $600 monthly, the chief of staff receiving $700, and also income from fees paid by nonmembers. In many instances, direct payments by patients constituted a substantial source of additional income.

Achievements.—The group practice prepayment plans have convincingly demonstrated that fairly complete medical care of high quality can be financed through prepayments at reasonable costs, provided that adequate facilities are supplied and the professional services are organized on the basis of group practice. The importance of these two prerequisites is fully confirmed by the experience of some industrial plans that are supported by company funds.[16] The feasibility and value of cooperative ownership of medical centers, such as hospitals and clinics, has been proved by the consumer-sponsored organizations. These alone are significant contributions to future planning, but there are more.

With few exceptions the scope of the provisions is broad, including preventive measures and treatment of the sick, professional and hospital services, and care at the home, the clinic, and the general hospital. There is continuity of service in health, acute sickness, and convalescence, although not through the whole period of long-term illness, and ready access to all types of available services with no regard to the total number or costs.

Preventive medicine, the touchstone of progress in medical care, is promoted by making health conservation an integral part of the programs and encouraging early diagnosis and prompt treatment. The plans refuse to draw an artificial dividing line between examination of the healthy and treatment of the sick, between professional advice and restoration of health. Comprehensive in service as they are, they can offer complete physical examinations, observe border-line conditions, detect incipient stages, and ensure early treatment. Thus they are able to minimize the incidence and severity of chronic illness.

The amount of care received by plan members compares favorably with that in other families. The majority of all subscribers up to 1945 had family incomes of less than $3,000. But the number of physicians' services at the home and clinic in this group equaled the rate previously observed in the general population among persons with family income of $10,000 or more. The frequency of care in general hospitals and the average number of days of hospitalization were about the same as among families earning $5,000 and more.

The exclusion of nonmedical practitioners from the staffs serves to maintain high standards of service. Apart from this a number of plans have made great strides in improving the quality of medical care. They have appointed well-trained and experienced physicians and members of related professions and developed well-equipped facilities for the care of the healthy and the ambulatory sick. They own or have ready access to hospitals meeting standards of adequacy, vest professional persons with full authority for all professional matters, see to it that ability and experience of the staff members are matched by intensity of effort in the performance of service, and stimulate postgraduate study. The patients and the physicians can easily and conveniently obtain the diagnostic services, consultations, specialist services, and special types of treatment so necessary to the practice of good medicine. The employment of auxiliary personnel not only relieves the physicians and dentists of time-consuming and annoying jobs but helps the patients to receive all the attention they need.

Encouragement of research is another distinctive feature of the plans. The Permanente Foundation, for instance, spent nearly $50,000 for this purpose in two years.[17]

The physicians and other professional personnel are benefited professionally and financially. Both general practitioners and specialists can realize their ideal possibilities, as they are offered scope and opportunity for close cooperation. The general practitioners are given the place they deserve rather than being relegated to the background or regarded as subordinates feeding business to specialists. The net incomes of the staff members compare favorably with those of physicians in individual practice, and the provisions for economic security are additional advantages of considerable value.

The total cost of the services are within the reach of a substantial proportion of the self-supporting people but are still too high to be afforded by families with limited resources or unstable income. They are much lower than those of individual practice fee-for-service plans with similar scope, because the economies afforded by the method of group practice are passed on to the "consumers" and the extra charges are fixed and relatively small. The total amounts of money annually expended by subscribers to group practice prepayment plans would buy but a fraction of the services actually received if care had to be procured without organized plan and paid for on a fee-for-service basis.

The principle of democratic control of the administration has been successfully applied by the cooperative health associations and the organizations which are cooperative in fact although not in name.

Shortcomings.—There are marked differences between the plans in regard to scope and quality of service, staff organization, and administrative structure.

A few organizations exclude hospitalization from their services, as they have encountered great difficulties in obtaining access to an adequate hospital in the community or in raising the funds for their own facilities. Nearly all disregard psychiatric service.

Some staffs do not measure up to high standards. These units have been unable to attract competent physicians, dentists, nurses, technicians, and others because the controversies over the combination of group practice and group prepayment have deterred well-qualified professional persons from affiliation. In some instances, mistakes in staff organization, in particular the failure to stress professional balance and divide authority among persons of equal rank, have led to quarrels, the formation of warring factions, and the loss of highly experienced physicians. The reluctance of some private medical groups to extend partnership rights to all staff members after a period of probation and the wide spread between the highest and lowest incomes of regular staff members have caused dissatisfaction.

The exclusion of subscribers from participation in the management of certain organizations, especially those owned by physicians in private practice and industrial companies, has alienated the persons who by their payments support the plans and, in addition, made it hard to foster the sense of responsibility so necessary to successful operation of any organization applying the principle of insurance.

The development of standards for group practice units is still in the stage of infancy, although repeated efforts have been made to formulate minimum requirements.

The total number of both organizations and subscribers is relatively small. "Additional stimulus is necessary if prepaid medicine is to be extended by this pattern." [18]

A challenging task lies ahead for medical statesmen: the formulation of principles for the sound organization and administration of group practice prepayment plans and the recommendation of legislation for the incorporation of such organizations.

NINE

Limitations and Potentialities of Voluntary Plans

THE remarkable increase in the number of participants in voluntary medical care insurance plans since the thirties has kindled high hopes. Continued expansion of such programs will ultimately bring adequate medical care of reasonable cost within the reach of all self-supporting people wherever they live, so the public is assured. All that is needed is time for development.

In every field of social venture it is evidence of actual achievements rather than good intention or enthusiastic pleading that prove the value of the undertaking. Voluntary medical care insurance is no exception to this rule. It is amenable to systematic inquiry and appraisal because it has a long record replete with all the facts necessary for proper evaluation.

In many foreign countries voluntary medical care insurance combined with disability insurance has been utilized for centuries. The reports on its achievements and shortcomings fill volumes. In the United States the first experiments were made in the nineteenth century, and the revival of the method began at the end of the third decade of the twentieth century without substantial modification of the basic patterns set before. It is of more than historic interest to compare the organization of European plans in the second half of the nineteenth century with that of American plans in the forties of the twentieth century. There is a close similarity in general policies, extending even to such questions as restrictions. To give one example only, the "Meyersche Kranken-Sterbe- und Unterstützungskasse für Berlin," a voluntary plan, according to its bylaws of

Limitations and Potentialities

1859 excluded from service those who had "a chronic disease or internal disorder found to be incurable," the mentally sick, and patients with venereal disease. Precisely the same clauses appear in many plans developed in the United States lately.

Mr. Gradgrind used to say, "What I want is facts." Facts and figures on the development and experience of the various types of voluntary organizations in the United States have been presented in Chapters Four to Eight. Impressive indeed are the lessons learned by trial and error in establishing and operating medical care insurance plans in this country. They are all the more significant as they confirm essentially what has been found in a score of foreign countries in more than one hundred years of large-scale experimentation.

Voluntary medical care insurance is of limited applicability in urban as well as rural districts. It holds considerable promise for development in industrialized areas with high purchasing power. These are the cardinal facts discovered long ago and rediscovered, tested, and verified time and again.

Before elaborating on the limitations and potentialities of voluntary plans, it is necessary to discuss the methods employed for their measurement.

METHODS OF MEASUREMENT

The factual knowledge which is the key to the evaluation of voluntary medical care insurance may be obtained in various ways. Intensive field studies of plans of various types may be made or pertinent information may be gathered by questionnaires. Material published in folders, bylaws, and annual reports may be analyzed. Statistical data on plans similar in type of provisions and method of organization may be collected, computed, and studied. The opinions of the people receiving service, of the participating professional persons and hospitals, and of the administrators may be ascertained by personal interviews or correspondence.

In actual practice all these methods have been employed

separately or in varying combinations. The best results can be expected from the combination of systematic field studies of representative organizations, personal interviews, and analyses of basic statistical data regularly reported by all plans.

The subject matter to be investigated is vast and lends itself to innumerable special studies. For the purpose of appraising individual plans and groups of similar plans, information must be assembled that answers at least the following fourteen questions:

1. Is the plan operated for profit or incorporated as a nonprofit organization?
2. Is the plan designed to pay cash indemnity or to render service in return for prepayments?
3. To what types of health conditions do the provisions apply?
4. What are the type, scope, amount, and duration of benefits or services?
5. What are the methods of organizing professional services, and what are the methods and rates of payment to the participating members of the professions?
6. What are the methods of organizing hospitalization and the methods and rates of payment to the participating hospitals?
7. What are the prepayment rates, extra charges for services, and additional obligations? Who bears the expenses and to what extent?
8. Where is administrative control vested, what is the composition of the administrative bodies, and what are their powers, duties, and functions?
9. What is the total number and the sex and age distribution of the persons enrolled at a given date?
10. What is the total number of participating professional persons, broken down by type of practice, and of beds in participating hospitals, broken down by type of service?
11. What is the number of eligible persons, by sex and age, who have received specified benefits or services during a certain period of time?
12. What is the number of specified benefits or services received by the eligible persons during a certain period of time?

13. What is the total earned income and the "other income" of the plan during a certain period of time?
14. What are the total expenditures for benefits or services and for administration, and what contingency reserves have been set aside during a certain period of time?

In evaluating the material assembled through the methods described before, including the systematic collection, proper classification, and correct computation of dependable statistical data, special attention must be given to the measurement of the services in regard to their quantitative and qualitative adequacy and of the costs in relation to both the average annual family income of the subscribers and the amount and quality of care received. The findings will show to what extent the plans encourage prevention of disease and promotion of good health, early diagnosis and treatment, and psychosomatic medicine; assure completeness, continuity, and consistency of service; improve the quality of medical care; and benefit the persons enrolled, the participating professional persons and hospitals, and the community as a whole.

LIMITATIONS

Voluntary medical care insurance can serve selected economic groups only. It can provide for limited services at reasonable cost but not for complete medical care if the plan is operated on the basis of the individual practice of medicine and the fee-for-service method of payment. These limitations are due to two main factors, psychological and economic.

All people who can afford regular prepayments for future medical care do not appreciate the advantages of insurance as protection against the economic hazards of sickness, injury, and maternity. Many self-supporting people refuse to participate in voluntary plans. Some, primarily those in the younger age groups, count on their previous good health record and are inclined to take care of today and let tomorrow take care of itself. Others consider illness a blow of fate, convinced that "fate will find a way," or share the opinion expressed in the following words: "If I am foolish enough to become ill I should pay for care just as if I am foolish enough to break a law and should pay the fine. The illness or punishment becomes more meaningful." Still others are uninterested in the proposition, doubting they will get their money's worth in their community or distrusting the promise of "complete protection against the full cost of care" printed in bold face in many folders, leaflets, and full-page advertisements. Thus voluntary plans have difficulty in attracting the very persons who because of their health status constitute favorable risks, and must expect to be swamped with applications from persons who are anticipating some service in the near future or have ailments which may require costly service.

The situation is complicated by the tendency of "favorable risks" to discontinue membership and of "poor risks" to remain faithful to the plan. Every year many subscribers cancel their membership, asserting they can see no profit in continuing their prepayments as they "did not have any sickness last year" or maintaining that the value of services received had been out of proportion to the amount of money paid into the pool. On the other hand, those who require or demand much service are most likely to continue their membership.

In short, the more favorable risks are slow to come in and quick to drop out, and the poorer risks are most anxious to join and stay. These psychological factors may easily lead to accumulation of less favorable, if not poor, risks and considerable financial difficulties or bankruptcy of the plan.

To minimize the danger ensuing from adverse selection of risks, voluntary plans cannot help but restrict both the freedom to join and the scope, amount, and period of the provisions offered. At least in their initial stage they must require group enrollment and insist on the participation of a certain percentage of all persons belonging to an organization, such as an industrial company, union, or association of farmers.

Limitations and Potentialities 193

They must limit eligibility to persons in certain age groups and refuse or restrict treatment for pre-existing conditions and specified diseases requiring much service.

Once a large membership has been built up, the voluntary plans can relax the eligibility requirements. Even then they cannot afford to open the door wide. But they are able to accept very small groups of employed persons and to offer individual enrollment subject to special conditions, such as the payment of higher rates or the absence of certain diseases and defects as certified by medical examination. They can extend or waive the age limit for group subscribers and maintain this policy as long as the proportion of older persons remains relatively low. In addition, they find it possible to liberalize their provisions by reducing the waiting periods for treatment of certain diseases, increasing the amount of benefits or services allowed, and extending the period for which subscribers are entitled to make claims. But they cannot operate successfully without many safeguards against the influx of unfavorable risks and heavy demand for service. Thus a large number of persons badly in need of protection and able to pay the average rates are barred from membership.

By force of circumstances, voluntary plans must give foremost consideration to the salability of their contracts and therefore set their prepayment rates low enough to make both benefits and price attractive to the public. But they must also make sure that the total earned income will be sufficient to cover the total current expenses and permit accumulation of contingency reserves.

In determining their rate structure, the plans must consider the principal factors bearing on costs: the scope and amount of the benefits or services offered in return for prepayments, the methods of organizing professional and institutional services, the methods and rates of payment to those rendering service, the need and demand for care on the part of the subscribers and their eligible family dependents, and the costs of acquisition and management. Control over the expenditures may be exercised by imposing restrictions on the benefits or by choosing that method of organization and payment for professional and institutional services which affords the greatest economies consistent with qualitative and quantitative adequacy of care. The expenses for promotion are always substantial and especially high in the first years, often absorbing as much as one third of the earned income.

Low prepayment rates within the reach of families with modest income yield funds sufficient only to finance very limited provisions. High prepayment rates producing enough money for comprehensive provisions defeat their own purposes because they can be afforded by a small fraction of the population only. The method of scaling the rates according to ability to pay is difficult to employ for voluntary plans.

The problem of establishing and maintaining a sound financial structure is especially serious if the plans are operating on the basis of the individual practice and the fee-for-service method of payment. It is much less grave for group practice plans, because the economies afforded by this method of organization can be passed on to the subscribers in the form of lower charges.

Voluntary plans are caught between the Scylla of prohibitive prepayment rates, supporting fairly complete service for the participants and adequate remuneration for those rendering care, and the Charybdis of low prepayment rates, covering very limited service and assuring the physicians and hospitals of reasonable payment. Even relatively inexpensive family contracts cannot be afforded by the large number of self-supporting families struggling to make ends meet and maintain the pride of economic independence, although they are ready to make some expenditures for medical care and are anxious to join a prepayment plan. If for the sake of argument the total average cost of a fairly comprehensive plan is estimated at $30 per person per year, a family of four would have

Limitations and Potentialities

to pay 4 per cent of an income of $3,000, 6 per cent of an income of $2,000 and 8 per cent of an income of $1,500.

In addition to psychological and economic factors, there are certain concepts which militate against the development of adequate programs on a voluntary basis. One school of thought holds that it is not the function of insurance as such to finance the small, easily anticipated expenses which create no economic hardship. This reasoning is often amplified by warnings of excessive demand that may be stimulated by an inclusive program. To prevent such happenings, restrictions, including deductible clauses, are frequently used. These "deterrents" are defended on the grounds that the patients can take care of the cost of trifling illness, that adjustment of small claims requires administrative costs out of proportion to the amounts involved, and that "patients will run to the doctor for every sneeze, sniffle, and headache. The doctor wouldn't be able to handle the load. Malingering will increase, and people will tend to become neurotic."

There is no fundamental reason why a program applying the principle of insurance should not include all the services needed for prevention and treatment. The problem is one of price rather than principle. With preventive services the costs of the plans will be temporarily higher at the beginning but markedly lower in later years. The objectives to be achieved are preservation and improvement of health and prevention of catastrophic illness by early diagnosis and early treatment of any condition that may result in serious illness. They can be attained only if the members of the prepayment plans have ready access to a well-rounded and well-balanced service. Those who favor deterrents to excessive use of a health program have failed to supply a satisfactory answer to the question: Who is to decide whether a condition is trivial or serious? The patient is no expert in diagnosis. If he were, he would not need a doctor. Quite justifiably the subscribers to a prepayment plan are anxious to obtain expert advice in regard to all their troubles. It is patently true that some patients ask queer questions, that some desire services which are unnecessary in the opinion of the expert, and that some—although very few—try to take undue advantage of the service. Without minimizing such possibilities, it cannot be stated too often that this problem must be solved by education and not by regimentation through contract clauses ruling out such and such service.

Many plans set income limits for enrollment or for provision of services covered by prepayments. This policy is advocated on the grounds that only persons with low income or only those below the "comfort level" need protection and should be entitled to subscribe or receive service. Acceptance of subscribers regardless of income would make further inroads in the incomes of physicians and other professional groups.

To make a just decision on the definition of the terms "low income" and "comfort level" requires the wisdom of a Solomon. How high or how low should the ceiling be set? Should it be designed to include or to exclude certain socioeconomic groups? There arise ticklish problems due to fluctuations of income within a short period of time, the difficulty of determining family income when several members are working, and the vast differences in the needs of the individual patients. "So many factors may enter the determination of income limits that the final result is seldom more than an arbitrary designation of a level high enough to include a substantial segment of the population." [1] Application of income limits is contrary to the basic principles of insurance because it may easily result in the insurance of many persons who constitute poorer risks, due to their socioeconomic and health conditions, and in the exclusion of the more favorable risks. It discourages families with several earners from enrollment, makes the proposition unattractive to management and labor because discrimination disturbs industrial relations, and breeds dissatisfaction—if not resentment—if it carries with it authority for the physicians to make additional charges. It results in the creation of two sys-

Limitations and Potentialities 197

tems, one for the "rich" who obtain the service they desire outside the plan and one for the "poor" who are eligible for such service as the plan provides.

At the risk of laboring the obvious, it must be stressed that the members of the health professions and the hospitals, clinics, and related facilities should be assured of payment commensurate with the value of their services. The chances of guaranteeing an adequate income to those rendering service are considerably reduced by limiting enrollment in a medical care insurance plan to people with meager resources, as low per capita income of the plan nesessarily spells low rates of compensation. They are considerably enhanced by admitting applicants irrespective of their economic status and thus building up substantial funds. Moreover, the payments from well-organized prepayment plans are safe, while the collections in other practice rarely exceed 70 to 80 per cent of the charges.

Weaknesses in the administrative organization are quite common under the voluntary method. Multiple agencies, some local and some state-wide, may be established within the same political unit. Their basic services and their standards of operation are likely to differ greatly. Competition and high expenses for promotion and administration are certain under such conditions. Vested interests are created that cannot be dislodged later when better plans are under consideration. Thus the ground is prepared for the policy of opportunism rather than principle in the future. All the basic objections to voluntary programs were aptly summarized by a minority group of the Committee on the Costs of Medical Care as early as 1932.[2]

If all the well-established facts are considered, the idea of a nation-wide program of voluntary medical care insurance appears unrealistic. Voluntary plans can be established in every state, this is beyond question. But they cannot reach all the self-supporting people in all the communities. Nor can they be expected to attain uniformity of basic provisions and with it reciprocity and easy transfer of subscribers. As history shows, solidarity knows no boundaries in times of great disaster but tends to end at the state lines in periods of "business as usual."

POTENTIALITIES

The potentialities of voluntary medical care insurance lie in the extension of the cost-sharing principle to persons other than subscribers, to agencies, or to both and in the combination of group practice and group prepayment. The first procedure serves purely financial purposes. It involves a decision on the method of procuring sufficient funds for the initiation and operation of voluntary plans. The second policy is designed to improve the quality of medical care and reduce its cost. It requires the establishment of group practice units working from medical centers, such as clinics or hospitals.

It is generally recognized that voluntary medical care insurance plans need "a shot in the arm" to develop widely and safely. The high costs of initial organization must be met, and the current income must be rapidly brought to a level permitting operation without deficit.

Financial aid for the establishment of nonprofit plans may be sought from foundations, wealthy citizens, or governmental agencies, local, state, or federal. Supplementary funds for operation may be obtained from employers or from the general public through taxation.

Force of persuasion may be used to induce employers to make voluntary contributions toward the operating cost by sharing the prepayments. This approach may result in the enrollment of many of the regularly employed persons, provided all employers, not only the big ones, participate. But it leaves out the many millions of families and individuals below the comfort level who are self-employed, irregularly employed, or are living on income from savings or pensions. In actual practice great difficulties have arisen in making employer participation universal, and no helping angel has appeared to supplement the prepayments of those persons below the com-

Limitations and Potentialities

fort level who are not wage earners or salaried employees. Because of this experience, compulsion rather than moral suasion has been advocated as an essential aid to voluntary plans.

As summarized in an official document these proposals entail:

> *Compelling* the payment of taxes to be used as a direct subsidy to the voluntary insurance plans, or
>
> *Compelling* the payment of taxes to be used as a direct subsidy to the low-income person or family wishing to enroll in a voluntary insurance plan, and for automatic enrollment of the indigent, or
>
> *Compelling* the employer to pay about one-half of the premium for persons wishing to enroll in a voluntary insurance plan.[3]

The Blue Cross Commission of the American Hospital Association has gone on record in favor of "grants-in-aid to state-approved voluntary health programs which are also supported by regular contributions from the beneficiaries."[4] The National Grange in 1946 adopted a committee report urging "that where the rural people cannot afford to pay the total cost of adequate medical care, public or private funds be used to supplement what payment the individual or family can reasonably make."[5] The New York Academy of Medicine Committee on Medicine and the Changing Order recommended in 1947 "that financial aid from city, state, or federal funds should be made available to voluntary non-profit plans approved by the state health or welfare office to enable them to meet the costs of initial organization and to underwrite deficits for the early years of the plan's operation, until the plan can be self-supporting."[6] The bill introduced in the United States Congress by Senators Taft, Smith, Ball, and Donnell on February 10, 1947, contains a proposal to allot tax funds to the states for the "extension of medical care services" and to authorize them to make payments to "any voluntary health, medical, or hospital insurance fund, or other fund, operated not for profit, in behalf of those families and individuals unable to pay the whole cost of such services or insurance therefor." [7]

Proposals for legislation to subsidize the operation of voluntary medical care insurance plans have far-reaching implications. Determination of ability to pay the full cost of needed services presumes agreement on the definition of the term "ability to pay," and this is difficult to achieve. Unavoidably it requires a "means test" and the establishment of a vast, cumbersome, and costly administrative machinery for its application. An army of investigators is necessary to assemble the facts on readily available family resources, verify statements, evaluate the medical need in relation to the economic conditions of the family, determine by guesswork, bargaining, and compromise how much the family can pay, and recheck the financial conditions from time to time. A second army of clerks must be employed to handle the files of the tens of millions of applicants and the accounts of "active cases."

The larger the subsidies which the taxpayers are compelled to provide for the expansion and improvement of voluntary plans, the hazier the demarcation line between the voluntary and compulsory methods of raising the funds. The greater the number of nonprofit organizations exempt from common types of taxation, the more urgent the need of the communities for new sources of revenue, such as sales taxes, to offset the loss.

Unquestionably, voluntary medical care insurance can bring very limited benefits or services within the reach of a considerable fraction of the population. But in the long run the public will not be satisfied with prepayment plans which, laden with restrictions, meet only a part of its total medical care needs, call for substantial additional expenditures to cover all the costs of service required, and stop where the direst exigency begins. Nor can the physicians be expected to be content with plans which disregard preventive services for the apparently healthy, "do only half a job" for the sick, and impede the practice of psychosomatic medicine. Those who hope that voluntary medical care insurance is here to stay and do not want to see it blown away, like dust, by the wind of legislation are searching for a convincing answer to the crucial questions: Does the voluntary method lend itself to the attainment of bigger objectives by slow and gradual evolution? Can it provide fairly complete medical care of high quality for all self-supporting persons able and willing to pay a reasonable price?

To make financial arrangements for groups of subscribers and disburse funds to those rendering care is one thing, to provide for quality of service quite another. Adoption of a prepayment plan without simultaneous organization of professional and institutional services meeting high standards and without building a suitable and efficient administration merely perpetuates old evils. It might make poor medical care more easily available by precluding improvements in the practice of medicine, dentistry, nursing, and related professions. In the words of C.-E. A. Winslow, "We have no right to collect either tax money or insurance funds for medical care without due assurance that real value will be received." [8] There is grave danger of unconditional surrender to the forceful argument that protection against the economic hazards of ill-health is the one and only problem to be solved by prepayment plans.

Good medical care, as taught and practiced by the leaders of the professions, cannot be practiced out of the little black bag. It is not assured merely by exposure of patient to physician, application of technical procedures, or examination by different kinds of specialists who have little commerce with each other. To reap the full benefits that can be derived from the advance of scientific medicine and to make medical practice as effective as possible, two policies must be adopted by prepayment plans. Due consideration must be given to the selection of competent physicians, to the qualification of those rendering the services for which payment is claimed, and to supervision of the indication for and the quality of the services performed. Second, the systematic association of general practitioners with specialists and the close cooperation of the representatives of various medical specialties must be organized through development of group practice units in medical centers. All evidence points to the conclusion that this policy holds great promise for the improvement of the quality of medical care.

The general extension of group practice depends first of all on the availability of medical centers and the development of regional systems integrating the several types of facilities. Such a system includes a main hospital affiliated with a medical school in a large city, regional hospitals performing certain teaching functions, district hospitals located toward the periphery, and "public health and medical service centers" in outlying districts. The combination of hospital facilities with the housing of physicians' offices, clinics, and health departments deserves serious consideration, as the American Public Health Association has pointed out.[9] Gigantic is the task of financing the construction and equipment of the many additional facilities needed. But the problem is not only one of raising capital funds. Within a region the cooperation of all institutions meeting standards of adequacy must be obtained, and locally group practice units must be established in the required numbers.

The current tendency to confine the functions of a voluntary medical care insurance plan to financial arrangements reflects the spirit of a bygone era. To be truly useful, the method of insurance must be employed for the improvement of professional and hospital services. Only then will the people receive the best that medicine, dentistry, nursing, and the related professions have to offer in the prevention as well as the treatment of illness.

There is a unique chance for voluntary medical care insurance to make real progress within its natural limitations, to

Limitations and Potentialities   203

help tens of millions of self-supporting people develop the capacity and opportunity to lead personally satisfying and socially useful lives. It lies in the combination of group prepayment and group practice, wherever feasible, and in the inclusion of comprehensive professional services and hospitalization in one program.

Bibliographical Notes

1: THE PRINCIPLE OF MEDICAL CARE INSURANCE

1. Sir Edwin Arnold, *The Light of Asia*, London, 1879, pp. 73-74.
2. Seth Luther, *An Address to the Working Men of New England*, New York, 1833, p. 16.
3. I. S. Falk, Margaret C. Klem, and N. Sinai, *The Incidence of Illness and the Receipt and Costs of Medical Care among Representative Family Groups*, Committee on the Costs of Medical Care, Publication No. 26, Chicago, 1932, pp. 209-11.
4. Alfred Manes, "Insurable Hazards," *The Journal of Business of the University of Chicago*, XIV (January, 1941), 4.
5. Carl Binger, *The Doctor's Job*, New York, 1946, p. 19.
6. Medical Group Practice Council, *Solo or Symphony*, New York, 1946, p. 9.
7. Dean A. and Katharine G. Clark, *Organization and Administration of Group Medical Practice*, New York, 1941, p. 9.
8. Committee on Research in Medical Economics, *Group Medical Practice*, New York, 1940; Franz Goldmann, "Potentialities of Group Practice," *The Connecticut State Medical Journal*, X (April, 1946), 289-94.
9. *Medical Care for the American People*, Committee on the Costs of Medical Care, Publication No. 28, Chicago, 1932, p. 155.
10. Franz Goldmann, "Instruction in Social and Economic Aspects of Medicine," *Journal of the Association of American Medical Colleges*, XVI (September, 1941), 299-307; "Teaching Health Economics in Medical Schools—Content and Method," Conference on Preventive Medicine and Health Economics, September 30-October 4, 1946, Ann Arbor, Mich., *Proceedings*, pp. 173-76.
11. Roger I. Lee and Lewis W. Jones, *The Fundamentals of Good*

Medical Care, Committee on the Costs of Medical Care, Publication No. 22, Chicago, 1932, p. 3.

2: TRENDS OF DEVELOPMENT IN THE UNITED STATES

1. Henry Harris, *California's Medical Story*, San Francisco, 1932, pp. 114–15.
2. *Ibid.*, p. 112.
3. Daniel Levy, *Les Français en Californie*, San Francisco, 1884, p. 189.
4. Walter Basye, *History and Operation of Fraternal Insurance*, Rochester, New York, 1919, p. 71.
5. Walt Whitman, *Leaves of Grass*, Selected and with an Introduction by Christopher Morley, New York, 1940, p. v.
6. Pierce Williams, *The Purchase of Medical Care through Fixed Periodic Payment*, New York, 1932, p. 254.
7. Helen Hershfield Avnet, *Voluntary Medical Insurance in the United States: Major Trends and Current Problems*, New York, 1944, p. 3.
8. Louis S. Reed, *The Medical Service of the Homestake Mining Company*, Committee on the Costs of Medical Care, Publication No. 18, Chicago, 1932.
9. International Ladies' Garment Workers' Union, *Union Health Center 1913–1940*, New York, 1940; *Triennial Report 1944–1946*, New York, 1947.
10. Evans Clark, *How to Budget Health*, New York and London, 1933.
11. Committee on the Costs of Medical Care, Series of 28 publications, Chicago, 1932.
12. U.S. Public Health Service, *The National Health Survey 1935–36*, Collected Papers, Washington, D.C., 1945.
13. Dean K. Brundage, "A Survey of the Work of Employees' Mutual Benefit Associations," *Public Health Reports*, XLVI (September 4, 1931), 2102–19.
14. R. R. Sayers, Gertrud Kroeger, and W. M. Gafafer, "General Aspects and Functions of the Sick Benefit Organization," *Public Health Reports*, LII (November 5, 1937), 1567.
15. National Industrial Conference Board, *Studies in Personnel*

Policy, No. 9, Health Insurance Plans, A: Mutual Benefit Associations, 1938, p. 8.
16. National Association of Manufacturers, *Industrial Health Practices*, New York, 1941, p. 67.
17. U.S. Bureau of Labor Statistics, *Health-Benefit Programs Established through Collective Bargaining*, Bulletin No. 841, 1945, p. 1.
18. National Industrial Conference Board, *Studies in Personnel Policy, No. 10, Health Insurance Plans, B: Group Health Insurance Plans*, New York, 1939, p. 11.
19. National Industrial Conference Board, *Studies in Personnel Policy, No. 9, Health Insurance Plans, A: Mutual Benefit Associations*, 1938, p. 18.
20. I. S. Falk, Don M. Griswold, and Hazel I. Spicer, *A Community Medical Service Organized under Industrial Auspices in Roanoke Rapids, North Carolina*, Committee on the Costs of Medical Care, Publication No. 20, Chicago, 1932.
21. Bureau of Cooperative Medicine, *Medical Care in Selected Areas of the Appalachian Bituminous Coal Fields*, New York, 1939.
22. U.S. Bureau of Labor Statistics, *Beneficial Activities of American Trade-Unions*, Bulletin No. 465, Washington, D.C., 1928, pp. 3, 12.
23. Pierce Williams, *The Purchase of Medical Care through Fixed Periodic Payment*, New York, 1932, pp. 291–301.
24. "Union Health and Welfare Plans," *Monthly Labor Review*, LXIV (February, 1947), 191–92.
25. American Medical Association, "Proceedings of the San Francisco Session, 1946," *Journal of the American Medical Association*, CXXXI (July 20, 1946), 994–95.
26. Margaret C. Klem, "Recent State Legislation Concerning Prepayment Medical Care," *Social Security Bulletin*, X (January, 1947), 10.
27. Nathan Sinai, Odin W. Anderson, and Melvin L. Dollar, *Health Insurance in the United States*, New York, 1946, p. 50. Reprinted by permission of the publisher, The Commonwealth Fund, New York.

28. Michael M. Davis, "Health Insurance Plans Under Medical Societies," *Medical Care*, IV (February, 1944), 223.
29. Social Security Board (now Social Security Administration), *Prepayment Medical Care Organizations*, 3d ed., Washington, D.C., 1945, pp. 3, 5, 11–12.

3: ATTITUDES OF NATIONAL VOLUNTARY ORGANIZATIONS

1. "Legislating for National Health," *Public Health Nursing*, XXXIX (June, 1947), 329.
2. American Medical Association, "Proceedings of the Cleveland Session, 1934," *Journal of the A.M.A.*, CII (June 30, 1934), 2200.
3. American Medical Association, "Proceedings of the Atlantic City Session, 1935," *Journal of the A.M.A.*, CIV (June 29, 1935), 2364.
4. American Medical Association, "Proceedings of the Special Session, 1935," *Journal of the A.M.A.*, CIV (March 2, 1935), 751.
5. American Medical Association, "Proceedings of the San Francisco Session, 1938," *Journal of the A.M.A.*, CXI (July 2, 1938), 59.
6. American Medical Association, "Proceedings of the Special Session, 1938," *Journal of the A.M.A.*, CXI (September 24, 1938), 1216.
7. American Medical Association, "Proceedings of the Atlantic City Session, 1942," *Journal of the A.M.A.*, CXIX (June 27, 1942), 728.
8. "Constructive Program for Medical Care," *Journal of the A.M.A.*, CXXVIII (July 21, 1945), 883.
9. American Medical Association, "Minutes of the Annual Session of the House of Delegates, 1945," *Journal of the A.M.A.*, CXXIX (December 22, 1945), 1209.
10. "National Health Program of the American Medical Association," *Journal of the A.M.A.*, CXXX (February 23, 1946), 495.
11. American Medical Association, "Proceedings of the San Francisco Session, 1946," *Journal of the A.M.A.*, CXXXI (July 13, 1946), 913–14.

12. American Medical Association, "Reports of Officers," *Journal of the A.M.A.*, LXXXVI (March 20, 1926), 865.
13. American Medical Association, "Reports of Officers," *Journal of the A.M.A.*, CIV (May 4, 1935), 1614.
14. American Medical Association, "Reports of Officers," *Journal of the A.M.A.*, C (May 6, 1933), 1411.
15. American Medical Association, "Reports of Officers," *Journal of the A.M.A.*, CIV (May 4, 1935), 1614.
16. American Medical Association, "Proceedings of the Atlantic City Session, 1937," *Journal of the A.M.A.*, CVIII (June 26, 1937), 2219.
17. American Medical Association, "Proceedings of the Special Session, 1938," *Journal of the A.M.A.*, CXI (September 24, 1938), 1216.
18. "Constructive Program for Medical Care," *Journal of the A.M.A.*, CXXVIII (July 21, 1945), 883.
19. "National Health Program of the American Medical Association," *Journal of the A.M.A.*, CXXX (February 23, 1946), 495.
20. American Medical Association, *Economics and the Ethics of Medicine*, Chicago, 1935, pp. 45–46.
21. American Medical Association, Reports of Officers," *Journal of the A.M.A.*, LXXXVI (March 20, 1926), 865.
22. American Medical Association, *Principles of Medical Ethics*, Chap. III, Art. VI, Sec. 2.
23. American Medical Association, "Reports of Officers," *Journal of the A.M.A.*, CXVI (April 19, 1941), 1803.
24. "Group Health Plans: Some Legal and Economic Aspects," *Yale Law Journal*, LIII (December, 1943), 177.
25. Michael A. Shadid, *A Doctor for the People: The Autobiography of the Founder of America's First Cooperative Hospital*, New York, 1939.
26. American Medical Association *v.* United States, 317 U.S. 519 (1943).
27. "Association Activities: Action of the American Dental Association House of Delegates on the National Health Program," *The Journal of the American Dental Association and the Dental Cosmos*, XXV (December, 1938), 2038.

28. "Association Activities: American Dental Association Committee on the National Health Program," *The Journal of the American Dental Association and the Dental Cosmos*, XXVI (January, 1939), 126.
29. American Dental Association, *Programs for Dental Health*, Chicago, 1941.
30. American Hospital Association, Thirty-Fifth Annual Convention, *Transactions*, XXXV (1933), 737.
31. "American Hospital Association Establishes Principles for Medical Service," *Journal of the American Medical Association*, CXI (October 15, 1938), 1470.
32. American Hospital Association, Forty-First Annual Convention, *Transactions*, XLI (1939), 159–60.
33. American Hospital Association, Forty-Fourth Annual Convention, *Transactions*, XLIV (1942), 134.
34. National Grange, Seventy-Fourth Annual Session, *Journal of Proceedings*, 1940, p. 151.
35. National Grange, Seventy-Eighth Annual Session, *Journal of Proceedings*, 1944, p. 39.
36. National Grange, Seventy-Ninth Annual Session, *Journal of Proceedings*, 1945, p. 164.
37. National Grange, *Legislative Program 1947*, p. 7.
38. American Farm Bureau Federation, *Official News Letter*, XXV (December 25, 1946), 6.
39. Farmers Educational and Cooperative Union of America, Thirty-Third Annual Convention, *Official Minutes*, 1937, p. 30.
40. Farmers Educational and Cooperative Union of America, Thirty-Ninth Annual Convention, *Report* II (1945), 367.
41. American Federation of Labor, Fifty-Eighth Annual Convention, *Proceedings*, 1938, p. 148.
42. American Federation of Labor, Fifty-Ninth Annual Convention, *Proceedings*, 1939, p. 194.
43. American Federation of Labor, Sixtieth Annual Convention, *Proceedings*, 1940, p. 126.
44. Congress of Industrial Organizations, First Constitutional Convention, *Daily Proceedings*, 1938, p. 207.

45. Congress of Industrial Organizations, Second Constitutional Convention, *Daily Proceedings*, 1939, p. 138.
46. Congress of Industrial Organizations, Fourth Constitutional Convention, *Daily Proceedings*, 1941, p. 272.
47. Railway Labor Executives Association, *Labor and Transportation*, Washington, D.C., 1946, p. 28.
48. International Association of Machinists, Grand Lodge, Twenty-First Convention, *Proceedings*, 1945, p. 147.
49. Chamber of Commerce of the United States, *Social Security in the United States*, Washington, D.C., 1944, p. 7.
50. Personal communication from the National Association of Manufacturers.
51. *Ibid.*

4: CASH INDEMNITY PLANS

1. Estimate by the Life Insurance Association of America.
2. W. A. Milliman, "Insurance Carriers and Medical Care Plans," in Chamber of Commerce of the United States, *Health Insurance in America*, Washington, D.C., 1945, p. 40.
3. American Federation of Labor, *Health Benefit Plans by Collective Bargaining*, Collective Bargaining Series No. 1, 1946, p. 7.
4. John M. Brumm, "Health Insurance Plans Under Union-Management Agreements," *Labor and Nation*, III (January-February, 1947), 47.
5. W. A. Milliman, "Insurance Carriers and Medical Care Plans," in Chamber of Commerce of the United States, *Health Insurance in America*, Washington, D.C., 1945, p. 45.
6. American Medical Association, Council on Medical Service, *Voluntary Prepayment Medical Care Plans*, rev., Chicago, 1947, p. 89.
7. State of Ohio, *General Laws of 1941*, Sec. 669–718.
8. State of New Hampshire, *Laws of 1945*, Chap. 96, No. 1.
9. State of New York, *Laws of 1946*, Chap. 548, Sec. 1.
10. American Medical Association, "Proceedings of the San Francisco Session, 1946," *Journal of the A.M.A.*, CXXXI (July 13, 1946), 913.

5: NONPROFIT HOSPITAL SERVICE PLANS:
BLUE CROSS PLANS

1. "Recommended Principles for Hospital—Blue Cross Relations," *Hospitals*, XX (August, 1946), 83.
2. American Hospital Association, *Approval Program and Standards for Blue Cross Hospital Service Plans*, 3d rev. ed., Chicago, 1942, p. 3.
3. American Hospital Association, Committee on Hospital Service, *Standards for Non-Profit Hospital Care Insurance Plans*, Chicago, 1938, p. 5.
4. American Hospital Association, *Approval Program and Standards for Blue Cross Hospital Service Plans*, 3d rev. ed., Chicago, 1942, p. 7.
5. American Hospital Association, *Blue Cross Approval Program*, Chicago, 1946, p. 8.
6. "Report of Medical Service Board," *Bulletin of the American College of Surgeons*, XVIII (June, 1934), 3.
7. New York State Legislative Commission on Medical Care, *Medical Care for the People of New York State*, Albany, 1946, pp. 214–17.
8. "Number of Member Hospitals above 3,200, Survey Reveals," American Hospital Association, Blue Cross Commission, *Blue Cross Bulletin*, VIII (January, 1945), 6.
9. "Recommended Principles for Hospital—Blue Cross Relations," *Hospitals*, XX (August, 1946), 83–84.
10. State of Michigan, *Public Acts of 1939*, No. 109, Sec. 1.
11. Odin W. Anderson, *State Enabling Legislation for Non-Profit Hospital and Medical Plans*, 1944, University of Michigan, School of Public Health, Public Health Economics, Research Series No. 1, 1944, p. 11.
12. C. Rufus Rorem, *Non-Profit Hospital Service Plans*, Chicago, 1940, pp. 99–102.
13. "Recommended Principles for Hospital—Blue Cross Relations," *Hospitals*, XX (August, 1946), 84.
14. American Hospital Association, *Blue Cross Approval Program*, Chicago, 1946, p. 7.

15. Personal communication from Mr. Edgar H. Clapp, Assistant Director.
16. American Hospital Association, Blue Cross Commission, *Milestones with Blue Cross, Annual Report 1944–1945*, p. 29.
17. Lester H. Perry, "The Coordination of Medical and Blue Cross Plans," *Journal of the American Medical Association*, CXXVII (February 10, 1945), 321–25; Louis J. Reed and Henry F. Vaughan, Jr., "The Coordination of Medical and Blue Cross Plans," *Journal of the American Medical Association*, CXXVIII (May 5, 1945), 22–25.
18. American Hospital Association, *Blue Cross Approval Program*, Chicago, 1946, pp. 7–14.
19. American Hospital Association, Blue Cross Commission, *Experience of Blue Cross Hospital Service Plans*, Annually.
20. E. A. Van Steenwyk, "The Administration and Underwriting of Hospital and Medical Insurance," in Chamber of Commerce of the United States, *Health Insurance in America*, Washington, D.C., 1945, pp. 33–36.
21. "More than Half of Hospital Cases Surveyed Found to be Result of Three Conditions," American Hospital Association, Blue Cross Commission, *Blue Cross Bulletin*, VIII (Post Conference Issue, 1945), 10.
22. New York State Legislative Commission on Medical Care, *Medical Care for the People of New York State*, Albany, 1946, p. 230.
23. Michigan Hospital Survey, *Hospital Resources and Needs*, Battle Creek, Mich., 1946, p. 69.
24. American Hospital Association, Blue Cross Commission, *Blue Cross Bulletin*, IX (April, 1946), 10.
25. Personal communication from Mr. John A. McNamara, Director.
26. Personal communication from Mr. Edgar H. Clapp, Assistant Director.
27. C. Rufus Rorem, "Nonprofit Hospital Service Plans," *Medical Care*, I (April, 1941), 135.
28. Personal communication from Mr. Richard M. Jones, Director, Blue Cross Commission.

29. U.S. Senate, *National Health Program*, Hearings on S. 1606, Part Two, p. 961.
30. Roger I. Lee and Lewis W. Jones, *The Fundamentals of Good Medical Care*, Committee on the Costs of Medical Care, Publication No. 22, Chicago, 1932, p. 3.
31. Louis H. Pink, *The Story of Blue Cross*, Public Affairs Pamphlet No. 101, New York, 1945, p. 4.
32. C. Rufus Rorem, *Blue Cross Hospital Service Plans*, 2d ed., Chicago, 1944, p. 87.

6: NONPROFIT PHYSICIANS' SERVICE PLANS: BLUE SHIELD PLANS

1. State of Michigan, *Public Acts of 1939*, No. 108, Sec. 1.
2. *Acts and Resolves of Massachusetts*, 1941, Chap. 306 (General Laws, Chap. 176B).
3. State of New Jersey, *Laws of 1940*, Chap. 74, Sec. 2 and 3.
4. Commonwealth of Pennsylvania, *Acts of 1939*, No. 398, Sec. 2.
5. State of Minnesota, *Laws of 1945*, Chap. 255, Sec. 2.
6. California Supreme Court, 1 Civil No. 12, 764. Excerpt in "Court Holds C.P.S. Not Subject to Insurance Laws," *California Medicine*, LXV (September, 1946), 138–42.
7. American Medical Association, *Voluntary Prepayment Medical Care Plans*, Chicago, 1946, p. 11.
8. *Ibid.*
9. Charles G. Hayden, *Massachusetts Medical Service*, Boston, 1946, p. 25.
10. *Ibid.*, p. 10.
11. *Journal of the American Medical Association*, CXXXI (July 13, 1946), 913–14.

7: NONPROFIT PLANS COVERING PROFESSIONAL AND HOSPITAL SERVICES: INDIVIDUAL PRACTICE PLANS

1. U.S. Senate, *National Health Program*, Hearings on S. 1606, Part Four, p. 2130.
2. R. C. Williams, "Development of Medical Care Plans for Low

Income Farm Families," *American Journal of Public Health*, XXX (July, 1940), 727.
3. U.S. Department of Agriculture, Farm Security Administration, Office of the Chief Medical Officer (later Health Services Division), Annual Reports.
4. Franz Goldmann, "Medical Care for Farmers," *Medical Care*, III (February, 1943), 28.
5. Robert L. McNamara and A. R. Mangus, *Prepayment Medical-Care Plans for Low-Income Farmers in Ohio*, Ohio Agricultural Experiment Station, Wooster, O., 1944, pp. 9, 14, 19.
6. Franz Goldmann, "Medical Care for Farmers," *Medical Care*, III (February, 1943), 29.
7. U.S. Senate, *The Experimental Health Program of the United States Department of Agriculture*, Subcommittee Monograph No. 1, Washington, D.C., 1946.
8. U.S. Senate, *National Health Program*, Hearings on S. 1606, Part Three, pp. 1161, 1169–70, 1178–79.

8: GROUP PRACTICE PLANS

1. Eugene L. Bishop, "Medical Care at a T.V.A. Project," *Medical Care*, II (July, 1942), 247–53.
2. Clifford Kuh, "The Permanente Health Plan," *Industrial Medicine*, XIV (April, 1945), 261–70.
3. James P. Warbasse, *Cooperative Medicine*, 4th ed., New York, 1946, p. 47.
4. Personal communication from Dr. G. Halsey Hunt, U.S. Public Health Service.
5. State of New York, *Laws of 1947*, Chap. 721.
6. State of Washington, *Laws of 1947*, Chap. 268.
7. State of New York, *Laws of 1947*, Chap. 722.
8. Personal communication from Dr. G. Halsey Hunt, U.S. Public Health Service.
9. Michael Shadid, *Co-op Hospital Catechism*, rev. ed., Walla Walla, Wash., 1946.
10. Franz Goldmann, *Prepayment Plans for Medical Care*, New York, 1941, pp. 37, 42.
11. Barkev S. Sanders and Margaret C. Klem, "Services and Costs

in a Prepayment Medical Care Plan," *Medical Care,* II (July, 1942), 218–19.
12. Sidney R. Garfield, "First Annual Report of the Permanente Foundation Hospital," *Permanente Foundation Medical Bulletin,* II (January, 1944), 42; "Second Annual Report . . . ," *Permanente Foundation Medical Bulletin,* III (January, 1945), 40.
13. Franz Goldmann, *Prepayment Plans for Medical Care,* New York, 1941, p. 36.
14. Barkev S. Sanders and Margaret C. Klem, "Services and Costs in a Prepayment Medical Care Plan," *Medical Care,* II (July, 1942), 222.
15. Sidney R. Garfield, "The Plan that Kaiser Built," *Survey Graphic,* XXXIV (December, 1945), 480–82.
16. Franz Goldmann, "Medical Care in Industry," *Medical Care,* I (Autumn, 1941), 301–12 and II (January, 1942), 3–17.
17. Sidney R. Garfield, "Health Plan Principles in the Kaiser Industries," *Journal of the American Medical Association,* CXXVI (October 7, 1944), 338.
18. W. Palmer Dearing, "Medical Service Plans Across the Country," *American Journal of Public Health,* XXXVI (July, 1946), 772.

9: LIMITATIONS AND POTENTIALITIES OF VOLUNTARY PLANS

1. Charles G. Hayden, *Massachusetts Medical Service,* Boston, 1946, p. 14.
2. Committee on the Costs of Medical Care, Publication No. 28, Chicago, 1932, pp. 131–32.
3. New York State Legislative Commission on Medical Care, *Medical Care for the People of New York State,* Albany, 1946, p. 359.
4. U.S. Senate, *National Health Program,* Hearings on S. 1606, Part Two, p. 965.
5. The National Grange, Eightieth Annual Session, *Journal of Proceedings,* 1946, p. 181.
6. New York Academy of Medicine, Committee on Medicine and

the Changing Order, *Medicine in the Changing Order,* New York, 1947, p. 57.
7. U.S. Congress, Eightieth Congress, First Session, S. 545, Title II, Sec. 204 providing for amendment of The Public Health Service Act, Title VII, Sec. 712 (a), No. 4.
8. C.-E. A. Winslow, "Medical Care for the Nation," *The Yale Review, XXVIII* (March, 1939), 518.
9. "Medical Care in a National Health Program," *American Journal of Public Health,* XXXIV (December, 1944), 1254.

Index

Ability to pay, difficulty of determining, 196, 200
Accident, unpredictability and fear of, 4-6
Achenbach Memorial Hospital Association, 149
Adequacy of medical care, 10, 33 f., 201
Administration of voluntary plans, 23-27; centralization vs. decentralization, 24; democratic control, 25, 50, 126, 186; directors and other officers, 25; state supervision, 26; dual, 50; commercial group policies, 75; employee benefit associations, 80, 81, 83; medical-society sponsored organizations, 91; Blue Cross plans, 104-6, 112; Blue Shield plans, 120-22, 126; Farm Security Administration plans, 134-36; group practice plans, 159; weaknesses common, 197
Agriculture, Department of, plans initiated by agencies of, 130-47
Alabama, enabling legislation, 85
Allegheny Ludlum Steel Corporation, 47
Allis-Chalmers Mutual Aid Society, 43
American Cast Iron Pipe Company, 46
American College of Surgeons, endorsement of prepayment, 95
American Dental Association, basic principles for dental care program, 62
American Farm Bureau Federation, 64
American Federation of Labor, attitude, 65
American Hospital Association, enrollment in plans approved by, 54; attitude toward prepayment plans, 62-63; role in development of Blue Cross plans, 94-95, 97-113; commissions, 97, 98; approval system, 106; in favor of grants-in-aid to state-approved programs, 199
American Medical Association, enrollment in plans approved by, 54; attitude toward voluntary plans, 55-61; toward physicians' service plans, 55-58; toward hospital service plans, 58 f.; creation and purpose of Council on Medical Service and Public Relations, 56 (*see entries under* Council); attitude toward group practice, 59-61; Code of Ethics, 59; Principles of Medical Ethics, excerpt, 60; Supreme Court ruling against, 61; on cash indemnity, 56, 57, 92; on additional charges, 117; approval system, 57
American Nurses' Association, 55
American Public Health Association, 202
American Woolen Company, 73
Ancient Order of United Workmen, 37
Ansco Mutual Benefit Association, 44
Associated Hospital Service of New York City, 103, 104, 179, 180
Associated Medical Care Plans, 57
Associated Women of the American Farm Bureau Federation, 64

Ball, Senator, 199
Baylor University Hospital, 94
Benefits, cash indemnity plans, commercial, 71-73; employee associations, 78, 81, 82; medical-society sponsored plans, 87-90
Binger, Carl, 13
Blue Cross Commission, 94, 98, 100,

220   *Index*

Blue Cross Commission (*Continued*) 106; in favor of grants-in-aid to state-approved programs, 199
Blue Cross Hospital Service of Ind., 105
Blue Cross plans, 45, 48, 50, 53, 63, 92; covering cash indemnity for surgery, 84; basic principles, 93; history and trends of development, 94-97; enrollment, 95, 96; role of American Hospital Association, 97-113 (*see entries under* American Hosp. Assn.); legal aspects, 98-99; eligibility requirements, 99-101; illness covered, 101; services, 101-3; prepayment rates, 103-4; paying the hospitals, 104; administrative organization, 104-6; approval system, 106; experience, 106-9; achievements, 109-11; shortcomings, 111-13; cooperation with Blue Shield plans, 106, 119, 121; bibliography, 212-14
Blue Shield plans for physicians' service, 45, 83-92, 114-26; service plans, history and trends of development, 114 f.; legal aspects, 115; cooperation with Blue Cross, 106, 119, 121; eligibility requirements, 116-17; type of illness covered, 117; type and scope of service, 117-19; organization of professional and hospital services, 119; prepayment rates, 119; administration, 120-22; approval, 122; experience, 122-24; achievements, 124; shortcomings, 125; bibliography, 214
Boards of directors or trustees, 25; cash indemnity plans, 75; Blue Cross, 104, 106; Blue Shield, 120; Farm Security Administration plans, 134
Brattleboro, Vt., hospital service plan, 95
Buddha, 3
Business, *see* Industry

California, mutual benefit associations, 35 f.; two outstanding plans, 78-81; enabling legislation, 85
California Farm Bureau Federation, 69
California Physicians' Service, 114, 116, 118, 119, 120, 123, 125
Cash indemnity plans, principle, 9-12; classification, 52; purpose, 68; commercial insurance policies, 68-77; nonprofit plans in industry, 77-83; those sponsored by medical societies, 83-92; bibliography, 211
Cass County, Tex., rural health service plan, 147
Centralization of administration, 25
Central Professional Service Committee, Mass., 121, 122
Chamber of Commerce of the U.S., endorsed voluntary plans, 67
Chattanooga, Tenn., payments by city for Blue Cross services, 104
CIO, *see* Congress of Industrial Organizations
Clark, Dean A., and Katharine G., quoted, 14
Classification and membership of plans, 51-54
Cleveland Hospital Service Association, 96, 105, 108, 109
Coal Mines Administrator, 47
Colorado Hospital Service, 102
Colorado Medical Service, 121
Columbia Employees' Hospitalization Plan, Torrance, Calif., 80 f.
Commerce, plans endorsed by the U.S. Chamber, 67
Commercial companies, *see* Insurance companies, commercial
Committee on the Costs of Medical Care, 5, 42, 197
Committees, of Blue Cross plans, 105; of Blue Shield boards, 121
Community Health Center, Two Harbors, Minn., 149
Community Surgical and Medical Care Plan, Toledo, 84
Compensation of professional personnel, methods, 17-21; effect of insurance, 23
Compulsory employer participation and tax subsidies proposed, 199

Index

Compulsory health insurance, endorsed by labor, 65
Congress of Industrial Organizations (CIO), health cooperatives and national health program endorsed by, 65; agreements by members of, 47, 73
Consolidated Edison Employees' Mutual Aid Society, 43, 148, 155
Constructive Program for Medical Care, of American Medical Association, 56; restatement, 57
Contract practice, 46, 114
Cooperative Health Federation of America, 149
Cooperative Hospital Association, Amherst, Tex., 155
Cooperative ownership of hospitals and facilities, 50
Cooperatives, 148 f., 158; endorsed by CIO, 65; examples of group practice plans, 167-72
Cost-sharing principle, 7, 198 ff.
Council on Medical Service and Public Relations, American Medical Association, approval of plans, 92, 112, 129; functions, 56, 57

Dallas, Texas, hospital service plan, 94
Davis, Michael M., 51
Death benefits, 36, 37, 43
Decentralization of administration, 24
Delaware, enabling legislation, 85; Blue Cross members, 96
Democratic control, 25, 50, 112, 126, 138, 186
Dental profession, attitude toward prepayment plans, 32; basic principles of program, 62
"Deterrents" to excessive use of programs, 195
Detroit, Mich., payments by city for Blue Cross services, 104
Directors, *see* Boards
Disability insurance, 6; relation of medical care insurance to, 29 f.
Doctors, *see* Physicians; Professional personnel
Donnell, Senator, 199

Economic disaster as result of sickness, 4-6
Education, on medical care insurance, 27-29; trained personnel, 29
Eligibility requirements, of commercial companies, 70; of employee associations, 78, 80, 82; medical-society sponsored plans, 86; Blue Cross, 99-101, 111; Blue Shield, 116 f.; Farm Security Administration plans, 131; group practice plans, 152
Elk City, Okla., cooperative hospital, 158, 167 f.
Employees, mutual benefit associations, 36, 42, 44; nonprofit plans in industry, 67, 77-83
Employer cooperation and plans, *see* Industry
Endicott Johnson Corporation, 46
Ethical argument stressed in American Medical Association's stand on group practice, 59-61
Europe, comparison of plans with those in U.S., 51, 188 f.

Farmers, enrollment in Blue Cross, 107, 111; Farm Security Administration plans (*q.v.*), 130-44; experimental rural health programs, 144-47; use of supplementary public or private funds urged in behalf of, 199
Farmers Educational and Cooperative Union of America, 64
Farmers Home Administration Act, 130, 136, 144
Farmers' organizations, opinions about health insurance, 63-65; cooperation of commercial companies with, 69; Blue Cross enrollment through units of, 96
Farmers' Union Hospital Association at Elk City, group practice prepayment plan, 149, 154, 167-69; physicians remuneration, 183
Farm Security Administration, nonprofit prepayment plans, 130-44; eligibility requirements, 131; type of illness covered, 131; type and scope of service, 131-33; organization of professional and hospital services,

Farm Security Administration (*Cont.*) 133; of payment, 134; administration, 134-36; experience, 136-38; achievements, 138-41; shortcomings, 141-44; relation to experimental rural programs, 144-47
Fear of illness and economic disaster, 3-6
Fee-for-service compensation system, 17, 18, 119, 127
Flat-rate compensation system, 17, 19
Florida, Blue Shield plan, 116
Franklin General Benevolent Society, 36
Franklin Hospital, 36
Fraternal beneficiary societies, 37, 42
Free choice of professional personnel, principle of, 10, 15-17; under commercial policies, 74; employee benefit plans, 79, 81, 83; cash indemnity plans sponsored by medical societies, 90; hospital service plans, 93; physicians' service plans, 114, 119; comprehensive individual practice plans, 127; group practice plans, 153 f.
French Hospital, Los Angeles, 36
—— San Francisco, 36
F.S.A., *see* Farm Security Administration

Gates Mutual Benefit Club, 148, 155; group practice prepayment plan, 164-67
General Aniline and Film Corporation, 45
German General Benevolent Society of San Francisco, 36
Grange, *see* National Grange
Grants-in-aid to state-approved programs, 199
Grinnell, Iowa, hospital service plan, 95
Group enrollment, 41, 49, 192; Blue Cross, 99; Blue Shield, 116; comprehensive individual practice plans, 128; group practice plans, 152
Group Health Association of Washington, D.C., 149, 155, 160, 182; description, 169-72

Group Health Co-Operative of Puget Sound, 149
Group Hospital Service, St. Louis, 105
Group Hospital Service of Delaware, 84, 88
Group insurance, growing role in commercial policies, 69
Group practice, principle of, 12-15; free choice, 16 (*see also* Free choice); attitude of American Medical Association, 58, 59-61; potentialities that lie in combination with group prepayment, 198, 202-3
Group practice prepayment plans, history and trends of development, 148-50; legal aspects, 150-52; eligibility requirements, 152; type of illness covered, 152; type and scope of service, 153; organization of professional services, 153-57; of hospital care, 157; prepayment rates, 158; administration, 159; examples of industrial plans, 148, 160-67; of cooperatives outside of industry, 148, 158, 167-72; examples of physician-controlled plans, 149, 172-78; of community-wide plans, 149, 178-80; experience, 181-83; achievements, 183-86; shortcomings, 186; bibliography, 215
Group prepayment, principle, 7-8; potentialities that lie in combination with group practice, 198, 203
Groups, representation on board of directors, 25
Guatama Siddhartha, 3

Hawaii Medical Service Association, 129
Health insurance, term, 6
Health Insurance Plan of Greater New York, 149, 156, 157, 159, 178-80
Homestake Mining Company, 40, 46
Honolulu County Medical Society, 129
Hospital Care Association of N.C., 84
Hospital Care Corporation, Cincinnati, 105
Hospitals, care for members of prepayment plans, 21-23; effect of insur-

Index

ance upon income, 23; essential to success of insurance plans, 31; cooperative ownership of, 50; removal from list of American Medical Association, 61; American Hospital Association's basic principle for purchase of hospital care, 62; provisions of commercial policies for services, 74; of employee benefit associations, 79, 81, 82; of medical-society sponsored organizations, 88; objectives and basic policies of all service plans, 93; Blue Cross plans, 93-113; role of the American Hospital Association, 97 ff. (*see under above subentries*); Blue Cross payments, 104; physicians' service plans may not include hospitalization, 116; their arrangements for hospitalization, 119; disadvantage of separate organizations for medical and hospital services, 126; individual practice plans (*q.v.*) covering professional and hospital services, 127-47; organization of hospital care, group practice plans, 157; regional organization, 202; housing of offices of physicians, 202; inclusion of their services in one program, 203

Hospital Saving Association of N.C., 84

Hospital Service Association of New Orleans, 84

Hospital Service Association of Northeastern Pa., 107

Hospital Service Association of Toledo, 107

Hospital Service Corporation of Ala., 84, 89

Hospital Service Corporation of R.I., 102, 105, 107

Hospital Service of Calif., 84, 88

Hospital Service Plan Commission, 97; succeeded by Blue Cross Commission, 98

Idaho, North, 117, 119

Illinois, legislation, 151

Illness, unpredictability of, 3-6; predictability, 7; types covered by commercial companies' cash indemnity plans, 71; employee-benefit plans, 79, 82; by medical-society sponsored cash indemnity plans, 87; Blue Cross, 101; Blue Shield, 117; Farm Security Administration plans, 131; group practice plans, 152

Income tax, exemption from, 46, 98

Individual practice, principle of, 12 f.; cash indemnity plans, 68-92; physicians' service plans, 114-26; comprehensive plans sponsored by medical societies, 127-29; F.S.A. plans, 130-44; experimental rural health programs, 144-47; bibliography, 214

Industry, mutual benefit associations in, 36, 42, 44; early plans for protection of employees, 39; later developments, 43 ff.; company-financed plans, 46, 47, 73; plans endorsed by National Association of Manufacturers, 67; employers' administrative responsibility for commercial group insurance, 75; cash indemnity plans, 77-83; role in three representative plans, 78, 80, 81; companies utilizing group practice, 148; examples of plans, 160-67; goal of universal employer participation, 198, 199

Insurance, compulsory: labor unions' desire for, 65 f.; Union Oil Company plan, 78-80

—— fraternal, 37

—— state laws governing cash indemnity, 85

—— voluntary medical care: principle of, 3-34; need for, 4-6; definition and objectives, 6; prerequisites, 6-8; characteristics, 8; feasibility, 8 f., 198; cash indemnity and service plans, 9-12, 50, 52, 68-92; free choice, 10, 15-17, 74, 79, 81, 83, 90, 93, 114, 119, 127, 153 f. (*see entries under* Free choice); individual practice, 12, 127-47, 191; group practice, 12-15, 58-61, 148-87, 198, 202-3; hospital care, 21-23, 31, 202; effect on income of professions and hospitals, 23; administration, 23-27, 50, 197; education, 27-29; relation to disability in-

Insurance (*Continued*)
surance, 29 f.; to broad health program, 30-33; trends of development in U.S., 35-54; early phase, 35-41; mutual benefit associations, 35, 42; fraternal beneficiary societies, 37, 42; commercial insurance, 38, 43; industrial companies, 39, 43-46; labor unions, 40, 46; distinctive features of first and second phases, 40 f., 49-51; second phase, 41-51; factors that aroused public interest, 42; new organizations assuming responsibility for plans, 47 f.; enabling legislation, 48; classification and membership of plans, 51-54; attitudes of national voluntary organizations, 55-67; cash indemnity plans, 68-92; Blue Cross plans, 93-113; Blue Shield, 114-26; individual practice plans covering professional and hospital services, 127-47; group practice plans, 148-187; comparison of American with European experiments, 188 f.; methods of measurement, 189-91; questions requiring special attention in appraising plans, 190-91; limitations, 191-98; potentialities, 197-203; bibliography, 205-17; *see also entries under above subdivisions, e.g.,* Administration; Insurance companies, commercial; Legislation; *etc.*

Insurance companies, commercial: differences between nonprofit and commercial plans, 27, 49; early developments, 38 f.; later developments, 43; persons covered by commercial insurance, 53-54, 69-70; cash indemnity plans, 68-77; history: trends of development, 68; eligibility requirements, 70; type of illness covered, 71; type and scope of benefits, 71-73; professional and hospital services: premium rates, 74; administration, 75; experience, 75; achievements, 76; shortcomings, 77; problem of utilization of, by profession-sponsored plans, 92

Insurance department, state: supervision by, 26, 49, 116

Interbureau Committee on Post-War Programs, U.S. Department of Agriculture, 144

Intercoast Hospitalization Insurance Association, Sacramento, Calif., 84

International Association of Machinists, 66

International Ladies' Garment Workers' Union, 40

Iowa Medical Service, 118, 120

Jones, Lewis W., 33, 110

Kaiser industries, 148
Kansas, 116
Kansas Hospital Service Association, 105

Labor Health Institute, St. Louis, 47, 149, 155, 158, 159, 182

Labor unions, early benefit plans, 40; later developments, 46 f.; opinions about health insurance, 65 f.; administrative responsibility, 75

Lee, Roger I., 33, 110

Legislation, insurance plans subject to state laws, 24, 85 f.; early phase, 48; enabling acts for hospital service and physicians' service plans, 48 f.; endorsements by farmers' organizations, 64; by labor unions, 65, 66; legal basis of Blue Cross plans, 98; of Blue Shield, 115 f.; of group practice plans, 150-52; proposals for alloting tax funds to states, 199

Loos, H. Clifford, 172; *see also* Ross-Loos Medical Group

Los Angeles, mutual benefit associations, 36; group practice prepayment plan, 149, 155 f., 172-76

Louisiana, enabling legislation, 85
Louisiana Physicians' Service, 88
Luther, Seth, quoted, 3

Macy, Mutual Aid Association, 37
Marion County Medical Service, W. Va., 118

Massachusetts, Blue Cross members, 96; enabling act, excerpt, 115; special committees, 121

Massachusetts Hospital Service, 121
Massachusetts Medical Service, 114, 115, 117, 118, 119, 121, 122, 123
Medical and Surgical Care, Inc., Utica, N.Y., 83, 87, 88, 89, 90, 91, 102, 124
Medical care, adequacy of, 10, 33 f., 201
Medical centers, necessity for availability of, and development of group practice units in, 202
Medical profession, see Physicians; Professional personnel
Medical Service, Charleston, W. Va., 84
Medical Service Association, Durham, N.C., 84
Medical Service Association of Pa., 84, 87, 88, 89, 116
Medical societies, cash indemnity plans sponsored by, 83-92; physicians' service plans operated under auspices of, 114-26; comprehensive individual practice plans, 127-29
Membership of plans, 52-54, 69-70, 83, 96-97, 114, 128, 129, 130, 145-46
Meyersche Kranken-Sterbe-und Unterstützungskasse für Berlin, 188
Michigan, 1939 enabling act, excerpts, 99, 115; Blue Cross plan statistics, 108; barrier to group practice, 151
—— University of, Student Health Service, 150
Michigan Hospital Service, 102, 103, 107, 109
Michigan Medical Service, 114, 115, 119, 120, 121, 123; surgical certificate provisions, 118
Midwives, role reduced, 147
Milwaukee, Wis., 116
Milwaukee Medical Center, 149, 155
Miners, provisions for medical and hospital fund, 47
Minnesota, act of 1945, 116
Missouri Medical Service, 84, 87, 88, 91
Missouri State Medical Association, 84
Mutual benefit associations, pioneers, 35-37; growth and later development, 42 f., 44; plans in industry, 67, 77-83

National Association of Manufacturers, 43; endorsed voluntary health plans, 67
National Bituminous Wage Agreement, 47
National Conference Board, 45
National Farmers Union, 64
National Fraternal Congress, 37
National Grange, 96; attitude toward insurance plans, 63-64; use of supplementary private or public funds recommended, 199
National Health Program, American Medical Association, 59
National Health Program Committee, American Dental Association, 62
National Organization for Public Health Nursing, 55
National voluntary organizations, summary of statements officially adopted, 55-67; bibliography, 208-11
Nebraska Medical Service, 84
New Hampshire, legislation, 85, 152
New Hampshire-Vermont Physicians' Service, 84, 88, 89
New Jersey, laws, 152; excerpt, 115
New York Academy of Medicine, Committee on Medicine and the Changing Order, 199
New York City, Health Insurance Plan, 149, 156, 157, 159, 178-80
New York State, enabling legislation, 85, 98, 151; Blue Cross plan development, 97, 108
Nonmedical practitioners, 16, 184
North Carolina, enabling legislation, 85
North Dakota Physicians' Service, 120
Northern Pacific Beneficial Association Northern Pacific Railway Company, 37, 148, 154
Northern Permanente Foundation, 148
North Idaho District Medical Service Bureau, 117, 119
Northwest Community Hospital Association, 149
"Nursing in Prepayment Plans," 55

Ohio, law of 1941, 85
Ohio Medical Indemnity, Inc., 84, 90

Ohio State Medical Association, 84
Oklahoma, Cooperative and Benevolent Laws, 167
Oregon, medical society plans, 127-29
Oregon Physicians' Service, 128

Patient-physician relationship, 10, 11, 13; *see also* Free choice
Pennsylvania, act of 1939, 116
Pennsylvania Medical Service Association, 84, 87, 88, 89, 116
"Per diem" method of hospital-care payment, 22
Permanente Foundation Health Plan, 148, 182, 185
Personnel, *see* Professional personnel
Physicians, status under cash indemnity and service plans, 10, 11; quality of service, 10, 13, 33, 201; freedom of choice, 10, 15-17, 74, 79, 81, 83, 90, 114, 119, 127, 153 f.; values of the "single fallible physician," 13; of cooperation between specialists and general practitioners, 14; compensation, 17-21, 23; factors that influence distribution of, 32; reasons for dissatisfaction with early plans, 41; contract practice, 46, 114; monopoly for plans by medical profession, 49; number participating in plans, 53; recommendations of American Medical Association, 55-58; punishments, by the Association, of group practice leaders, 61; agreements made by medical-society sponsored organizations, 90; physicians on their boards, 91; payment under cash indemnity plans, 68, 74, 83, 90; value of Blue Cross plans to, 110; nonprofit service plans, 114-26; response to profession-sponsored cash indemnity plans, 85; Blue Shield plans, 124; effects of plans upon, 124, 125; individual practice plans covering hospital and professional services, 127-47; development and examples of physician-controlled group practice plans, 149, 172-78; legal basis of group practice prepayment plans, 150; organization of professional services in group practice plans, 153-57; combination of housing facilities of, with those of hospitals, 202; of comprehensive services and hospitalization in one program, 203; *see also* Professional personnel
Practitioners, nonmedical, 16, 184
Predictability of illness, 7
Premium rates, commercial companies, 74; *see also* Prepayment rates
Prepayment rates, employee benefit associations, 80, 81, 83; medical-society sponsored cash indemnity plans, 90; Blue Cross, 103 f.; Blue Shield, 119; Farm Security Administration plans, 134; group practice plans, 158; determination of rates: factors to be considered, 193 ff.
Preventive services, 125, 184, 195, 200
Principles of Medical Ethics, 60
Professional personnel, individual vs. group practice, 12 ff.; education, 29; adequate, in each service area, essential to success of insurance plan, 31; dental profession, 32, 62, 142; pooling of administrative personnel by medical society and hospital service plans in Mass., 121; necessity for assured and adequate compensation of, 197; *see also* Physicians
Psychosomatic medicine, practice impeded, 125, 201
Public Health Service, U.S., 42, 150, 154
Public health services, essential to operation of insurance plan, 30
Puerto Rico, payments by government for Blue Cross services, 104

Quality of service, 10, 13, 33 f.; 201
Queen of Angels Hospital, 175

Railway Labor Executives' Association, 66
Rates of payment for hospital care, determination, 22 f.; *see also* Prepayment rates
Rates of prepayment, factors bearing on, 193 ff.

Index

Regional hospital system, 202
Resettlement Administration, 130; see Farm Security Administration
Retail, Wholesale, and Department Store Union, CIO, 47
Rhode Island, Blue Cross plan, 96, 102, 105, 107, 109
Risks, favorable vs. poor: dangers ensuing from adverse selection, 192 f.
Roanoke Rapids, N.C., 45
Rockford, Ill., 95
Rorem, C. Rufus, quoted, 113
Ross, Donald E., 172
Ross-Loos Medical Group, 149; specialties represented on staff, 155 f.; group practice prepayment plan, 172-76
Rural Health Services Association, Newton County, Miss., 144
Rural plans, see under Farmers

Salary system of compensation, 18, 20
San Francisco, mutual benefit associations, 36
Sapulpa, Okla., payments by city for Blue Cross services, 104
Service plans, principle of, 9-12; development of, 50; classification, 52; position of American Medical Association, 56-57; of Blue Cross, 93-94; see also Hospitals; Physicians
Shadid, Michael A., 167
"Single-package plans," 127; see Individual practice plans
Smith, Senator, 199
Social Security Act, 98
Social Security Administration, study by, statistics, 53
Société Française de Bienfaisance Mutuelle, Los Angeles, 36
—— San Francisco, 36
Southern Pacific Company, 45
South Plains Cooperative Hospital Association, 149
Spaulding Employees' Mutual Benefit Association, 81-83
Specialists, see Physicians
Standard Oil Company of La., 45; see also Stanocola
Standard Railway Labor Unions, 65

Stanocola Employees' Medical and Hospital Association, 43, 45, 148, 154; specialties represented on staff, 155 f.; description of plan, 162-64
State Medical Society of Wis., 84
States, supervision of plans by, 24, 26, 49, 116; proposals to allot tax funds to, 199
Steel workers' program, 47
Supreme Court, ruling against American Medical Association, 61
Surgical-Medical Care, Kansas City, 120

Taft, Senator, 199
Taxation, exemption from, 46, 98; proposals for allotting tax funds for medical care, 199
Tennessee, legislation, 152
Tennessee Coal, Iron and Railroad Company, 45, 148, 154; group practice prepayment plan, 160-62
Tennessee Valley Authority, 148
Texas, consumer cooperatives, 149
Textile industry, findings of study, 75
Textile Workers' Union of America, CIO, 73
Trinity Hospital, Little Rock, 149; group practice prepayment plan, 176-78
Trustees, see Boards

Union Health Center, 40
Union Oil Company of Calif., Employees' Benefit Plan, 43, 44, 78-80
United Medical Service in New York City, 83, 86, 88, 89, 90
United Mine Workers, A F of L, 47
United Nations, 180
United States Public Health Service, 42, 150, 154
United Steel Workers of America, CIO, 47

Vermont, New Hampshire-Vermont Physicians' Service, 84, 88, 89
Veterans Administration, 121; Blue Cross plans utilized by, 105

Wagner-Murray-Dingell Bill, 65
Washington, medical society plans, 127-29; law of 1947, 151
Washington State Medical Bureau, 128
Western New York Medical Plan, Inc., Buffalo, 83, 124

Whitman, Walt, 39
Winslow, C.-E. A., quoted, 201
"Wisconsin Plan," 85
Workmen's Benefit Fund of the U.S., 38

Bei Fragen zur Produktsicherheit wenden Sie sich bitte an:
If you have any questions regarding product safety,
please contact:

Walter de Gruyter GmbH
Genthiner Straße 13
10785 Berlin
productsafety@degruyterbrill.com